Clinical Use of Neuroleptic Plasma Levels

Clinical Use of Neuroleptic Plasma Levels

Edited by
Stephen R. Marder, M.D.
John M. Davis, M.D.
Philip G. Janicak, M.D.

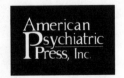

Washington, DC
London, England

Note: The authors have worked to ensure that all information in this book concerning drug dosages, schedules, and routes of administration is accurate as of the time of publication and consistent with standards set by the U.S. Food and Drug Administration and the general medical community. As medical research and practice advance, however, therapeutic standards may change. For this reason and because human and mechanical errors sometimes occur, we recommend that readers follow the advice of a physician who is directly involved in their care or the care of a member of their family.

Copyright © 1993 American Psychiatric Press, Inc.
ALL RIGHTS RESERVED
Manufactured in the United States of America on acid-free paper
First Edition
96 95 94 93   4 3 2 1

American Psychiatric Press, Inc.
1400 K Street, N.W., Washington, DC   20005

Library of Congress Cataloging-in-Publication Data
Clinical use of neuroleptic plasma levels / edited by Stephen R.
  Marder, John M. Davis, and Philip G. Janicak.
    p.   cm.
    Includes bibliographical references and index.
    ISBN 0-88048-524-8
    1. Antipsychotic drugs—Pharmacokinetics. 2. Antipsychotic drugs—
Dose-response relationship. 3. Blood—Analysis. I. Marder,
Stephen R., 1945–   . II. Davis, John M. (John Marcell), 1933–
III. Janicak, Philip G.
    [DNLM: 1. Tranquilizing Agents, Major—blood. 2. Tranquilizing
Agents, Major—therapeutic use.   QV 77.9 C641 1993]
    RM333.5.C45   1993
    616.89′18—dc20
DNLM/DLC
for Library of Congress   93-16126
                                                                                                    CIP

British Library Cataloguing in Publication Data
A CIP record is available from the British Library.

Contents

Contributors vii

Introduction xi
    Stephen R. Marder, M.D., John M. Davis, M.D., and
    Philip G. Janicak, M.D.

1. Neuroleptic Plasma Levels: Limitations and Values 1
    Bruce M. Cohen, M.D., Ph.D., and Christine Waternaux, Ph.D.

2. Neuroleptic Plasma Levels: Methodological Issues,
Study Design, and Clinical Applicability 17
    Philip G. Janicak, M.D., Javaid I. Javaid, Ph.D., and
    John M. Davis, M.D.

3. Fluphenazine Plasma Levels, Dose, and Acute
Treatment Response 45
    Douglas F. Levinson, M.D., George M. Simpson, M.D.,
    E.-S. Lo, Ph.D., and Thomas B. Cooper, M.A.

4. Haloperidol Plasma Levels and Clinical Response 63
    Theodore Van Putten, M.D., and Stephen R. Marder, M.D.

5. Haloperidol Plasma Levels and Initial Response to
Neuroleptic Treatment 77
    John M. Davis, M.D., Stephen E. Ericksen, M.D.,
    Stephen Hurt, Ph.D., Sidney S. Chang, M.D.,
    Javaid I. Javaid, Ph.D., Haroutune Dekirmenjian, Ph.D., and
    Regina Casper, M.D.

6. Clinical Use of Clozapine Plasma Concentrations 85
    Paul J. Perry, Ph.D., and Del D. Miller, Pharm.D., M.D.

7. Plasma Level Monitoring for Long-Acting
Injectable Neuroleptics 101
  Stephen R. Marder, M.D., Theodore Van Putten, M.D.,
  Manickam Aravagiri, Ph.D., William C. Wirshing, M.D., and
  Kamal K. Midha, D.Sc.

8. Neuroleptic Plasma Concentrations: An Estimate of Their
Sensitivity and Specificity as a Predictor of Response 113
  Paul J. Perry, Ph.D., and Daniel A. Smith, Pharm.D.

9. Use and Interpretation of Neuroleptic Plasma Levels 137
  Stephen R. Marder, M.D., John M. Davis, M.D., and
  Philip G. Janicak, M.D.

Index 143

Contributors

Manickam Aravagiri, Ph.D.
Assistant Research Pharmacologist, University of California at Los Angeles School of Medicine, Los Angeles, California

Regina Casper, M.D.
Professor, Department of Psychiatry and Behavioral Sciences, Stanford University School of Medicine, Stanford, California

Sidney S. Chang, M.D.
Director, Inpatient Psychiatry, Brockton Veterans Affairs Medical Center; Assistant Professor, Department of Psychiatry, Harvard Medical School, Boston, Massachusetts

Bruce M. Cohen, M.D., Ph.D.
Associate Professor of Psychiatry, Harvard Medical School, Boston; McLean Hospital, Belmont, Massachusetts

Thomas B. Cooper, M.A.
Associate Professor of Psychopharmacology in Psychiatry, Columbia University, Nathan Kline Institute, Orangeburg, New York; New York State Psychiatric Institute, New York, New York

John M. Davis, M.D.
Gilman Professor of Psychiatry, University of Illinois at Chicago; Chief, Research Unit, Illinois State Psychiatric Institute, Chicago, Illinois

Haroutune Dekirmenjian, Ph.D.
National Psychopharmacology Laboratory, Knoxville, Tennessee

Stephen E. Ericksen, M.D.
University of California, Davis Medical Center, Sacramento, California

Stephen Hurt, Ph.D.

Associate Professor of Clinical Psychology in Psychiatry, Cornell University Medical Center, Westchester Division, White Plains, New York

Philip G. Janicak, M.D.

Professor of Psychiatry, University of Illinois at Chicago; Director of Research, Illinois State Psychiatric Institute, Chicago, Illinois

Javaid I. Javaid, Ph.D.

Associate Professor of Psychiatry, University of Illinois at Chicago, Chicago, Illinois

Douglas F. Levinson, M.D.

Associate Professor of Psychiatry, Medical College of Pennsylvania; Eastern Pennsylvania Psychiatric Institute, Philadelphia, Pennsylvania

E.-S. Lo, Ph.D.

Associate Research Professor of Psychiatry, College of Physicians and Surgeons, Columbia University; New York State Psychiatric Institute, New York, New York

Stephen R. Marder, M.D.

Professor of Psychiatry, University of California at Los Angeles School of Medicine; Chief, Psychiatry Service, West Los Angeles Veterans Affairs Medical Center, Los Angeles, California

Kamal K. Midha, D.Sc.

Professor of Pharmacy, College of Pharmacy, University of Saskatchewan, Saskatoon, Canada

Del D. Miller, Pharm.D., M.D.

Professor of Pharmacy, College of Medicine, University of Iowa, Iowa City, Iowa

Paul J. Perry, Ph.D.

Professor of Psychiatry and Professor of Pharmacy, College of Medicine, College of Pharmacy, University of Iowa, Iowa City, Iowa

Contributors

George M. Simpson, M.D.

Professor of Psychiatry, Medical College of Pennsylvania; Eastern Pennsylvania Psychiatric Institute, Philadelphia, Pennsylvania

Daniel A. Smith, Pharm.D.

Adjunct Clinical Assistant Professor of Pharmacy, College of Pharmacy, College of Medicine, University of Iowa, Iowa City, Iowa

Theodore Van Putten, M.D.

Professor of Psychiatry, University of California at Los Angeles School of Medicine; Brentwood Division, West Los Angeles Veterans Affairs Medical Center, Los Angeles, California

Christine Waternaux, Ph.D.

Assistant Professor of Biostatistics, Harvard Medical School, Harvard School of Public Health, Boston; McLean Hospital, Belmont, Massachusetts

William C. Wirshing, M.D.

Adjunct Assistant Professor of Psychiatry, University of California at Los Angeles School of Medicine; Brentwood Division, West Los Angeles Veterans Affairs Medical Center, Los Angeles, California

CHAPTER 1

Neuroleptic Plasma Levels: Limitations and Values

Bruce M. Cohen, M.D., Ph.D.
Christine Waternaux, Ph.D.

T he study of drug levels in blood in patients and animals has allowed key parameters of absorption, metabolism, distribution, and elimination to be defined for numerous medications. Knowing these parameters has been essential for designing and interpreting studies of drug actions. However, determining the concentration of drugs in blood is not a procedure routinely used to monitor clinical treatment with most medications. For many drugs, assays are not available or reliable. For others, blood levels have little relationship to clinical effects because the concentration of drug in blood does not correlate highly with the concentration of drug at major sites of action or because there is no simple mechanistic relationship between drug concentration and drug effects (Cohen 1984).

For neuroleptic antipsychotic drugs especially, there have been special reasons to hope that blood levels would be predictive of outcome so that determining blood levels would improve treatment. Unlike many medications, the clinical effects of antipsychotic drugs are slow to develop, and it can be days to weeks between the onset of treatment and the appearance of therapeutic benefit (Cohen 1988; Keck et al. 1989). Maximal therapeutic and side effects (notably the onset of tardive dyskinesia) can be delayed

This material was presented in part at a symposium on "The Clinical Utility of Neuroleptic Drug Levels" at the 143rd Annual Meeting of the American Psychiatric Association, New York, May 1990. We thank Rebecca Thompson for preparation of this manuscript. This work was supported in part by Public Health Service grants MH31154, MH38313, MH42543, and MH43679 and gifts from E. I. duPont de Nemours and Company and the Kali-Duphar Laboratories.

even longer. Any procedure that could identify an optimal drug regimen earlier in treatment would save considerable time in trial-and-error dose adjustments and, thereby, considerable suffering and expense.

If dose were strongly correlated with clinical outcome, there would be far less interest in the study of blood levels of neuroleptics. However, dose is only a weak predictor of the therapeutic effects of antipsychotic drugs (Cohen 1988; Baldessarini et al. 1988). This may be in part because of the large differences that exist between individuals in absorption and metabolism of neuroleptics and, as a consequence, low correlations between the drug given and the drug found in tissue (Cohen 1984). Measuring neuroleptic levels directly in blood may partially obviate these differences and might lead to better predictability of short- and long-term therapeutic and toxic effects.

Problems in Interpreting Blood Levels of Neuroleptics

Unfortunately, although the blood level of a drug might be a better predictor of outcome than dose, there is little reason to believe that the predictive value of neuroleptic blood levels will be high.

1. Although blood levels can account for interindividual differences in drug absorption from gut to blood, they cannot account for differences in distribution from blood to brain that are dependent on variables such as protein binding and the relative lipophilic qualities of specific drugs. Like absorption, distribution of neuroleptics varies widely among drugs and may vary between individuals, which would obscure the relationship between drug levels in blood and effects in the brain (Sunderland and Cohen 1987).

2. Neuroleptics appear to concentrate markedly in cell membranes near the monoamine receptors through which they act (Cohen and Zubenko 1985a). Their concentrations at these sites may not be equal to drug levels in brain, let alone in blood (Cohen 1984). Therefore, the level of a drug in blood may bear no constant relationship to its level at the site of action.

3. Metabolites are believed to be important in determining the actions of neuroleptic antipsychotic drugs, and measuring concentrations of the parent drug alone may provide a poor estimate of the drug's activity in the blood or brain (Cohen et al. 1979). However, the existence of key

metabolites may be unknown. In addition, because the relative potency and distribution of metabolites is not well documented, the contribution of metabolites to clinical drug effects is difficult to assess.

4. The delayed therapeutic effects of neuroleptics suggest that the direct actions of these agents are only the first step in a cascade of changes that lead to the eventual drug-induced reduction of psychotic symptoms. There may be no simple or direct relationship between neuroleptic levels, even at their active sites, and the long-term effects of neuroleptics.

5. Sensitivity to drugs may vary markedly between individuals (Cohen and Zubenko 1985b). These interindividual differences in responsiveness rather than differences in drug levels may be the greatest determinant of therapeutic outcome.

6. If implications can be drawn from animal models, it is probable that even in a particular individual tissue sensitivity to drug changes with time of day and season (Campbell et al. 1982). In addition, tissue sensitivity and response to drug changes with time following administration (Cohen et al. 1991; Clow et al. 1980). Thus the same dose or tissue concentration of a drug will have different effects even in the same patient at different times during treatment.

In summary, drug levels measured in blood may be weak predictors of neuroleptic concentration at the site of action. In addition, drug concentrations at key sites may be only weakly predictive of long-term effects, whereas the relationship of level to effect may differ widely from one patient to the next or even in the same patient over time. For these reasons, expectations about the degree of correlation of drug levels to drug effects should be modest.

Correlation of Neuroleptic Levels to Drug Effects

Although it is important to temper our expectations of the value of a neuroleptic level, the degree of correlation between blood levels and effects must ultimately be determined by experiment. Over time, many studies have attempted to determine this relationship. However, meaningful studies have not been easy to perform because of methodological requirements. These requirements have been extensively reviewed elsewhere (Davis et al. 1978; May et al. 1981; Cohen 1984) but briefly are as follows.

3

The patients studied must have disorders that are likely to be drug responsive; typically this means they should be acutely psychotic or in an acute exacerbation of a chronic psychotic illness. Homogeneity of illness may be important although there is little evidence that patients with different diagnostic subtypes of psychotic illness respond differently to medication when their illness has acutely worsened. Neuroleptic doses must be predetermined and fixed during the period of study and patients must be randomly assigned to a dose so as not to confound dose selection and concomitant drug level with severity of presentation or early signs of response. Low and moderate doses must be included to observe the upswing of a curve relating dose or blood level to response. Patients must be studied on fixed doses (or levels) of drug for an adequate period of time for an antipsychotic effect to be observed. This requires more than a week of treatment. Valid and appropriate assays must be available for substances (both parent drug and active metabolites) of interest. Similarly, measures of clinical state (symptoms and side effects) must be sensitive, reliable, and valid and must be completed by individuals blind to drug doses and blood levels.

Few studies have incorporated all of these features. For our review at the 1990 Annual Meeting of the American Psychiatric Association (May 1990), we collected studies that satisfied the criteria of enrolling patients with acute psychosis or an acute exacerbation of psychosis, and employed fixed, predetermined doses of antipsychotic drugs for at least 2 weeks. These studies are listed in Table 1–1. The list is not comprehensive because no computer search of the literature was performed and no studies are included that were published after the time of our presentation.

For these studies, we have listed the drug, dose, and number of subjects and noted the kind of correlation observed between drug levels and effects. Where possible, we calculated R (a measure of correlation between blood levels and clinical outcome, with R^2 being the proportion of outcome variance accounted for by differences in blood levels of drug).

With even a quick overview, it is evident that study design and outcome were highly variable. There are few studies of most drugs and the studies used different patient populations, drug doses, and assays even when the same drug was chosen. Not surprisingly, a wide range of findings were observed. In fact, among individual studies it is possible to find representatives of all possible associations between blood levels and drug effects, from positive to negative correlations and from strong correlations to no or weak correlations. Also, among significant correlations of blood levels to drug effects, both linear and curvilinear relationships were reported. The curvilinear relationships observed were often so-called inverted U shape in

Table 1–1. Fixed-dose studies of the correlation of plasma concentration of neuroleptics and clinical response

Drug	Study	Dose (mg/day)	N subjects	R
Haloperidol	Bigelow et al. (1985)	~28	19	.12(L)
	Bleeker et al. (1984)	5–10	29	.01(L)
	Contreras et al. (1987)	20–40	27	.04(L)
	Garver et al. (1984)	6–24	17	Yes (C)
	Greenberg et al. (1983)	10–30	11	Yes (L)
	Kirch et al. (1988)	~28	30	-.03(L)
	Linkowski et al. (1984)	30	30	.42(C)
	Mavroidis et al. (1983)	3–12	14	.66(C)
	Potkin et al. (1985)	~28	43	.28(L)
	Santos et al. (1989)	15–30	24	.69(C)
	Shostak et al. (1987)	10	17	.19(L)
	Smith et al. (1985a, 1985b)	10–20	33	.34(C)
	Smith (1987)	8–40	24	.04(C)
	Tang et al. (1984)	60	19	.28(L)
	Van Putten et al. (1985)	5–20	76	.40(C)
	Wistedt et al. (1984)	15	10	.62(L)
Chlorpromazine	Alfredsson et al. (1985)	800	25	No
	Clark et al. (1978)	300–900	25	No
	Lader (1976)	300	32	.32(L)
	May et al. (1981)	450	48	No
	Sakalis et al. (1972)	300	10	No
	Wode-Helgodt et al. (1978)	200–600	38	.28(L)
Fluphenazine	Dysken et al. (1981)	5–20	29	.53(L)
	Hitzeman et al. (1986)	5–20	15	No
	Mavroidis et al. (1984)	5–20	19	.47(C)
Thioridazine	Cohen et al. (1989a)	200–400	53	.22(C)
	Smith et al. (1984)	150–750	26	.11(L)
Thiothixene	Mavroidis et al. (1984a, 1984b)	8–30	14	.60(C)
	Van Putten et al. (1983)	~30	34	.29(L)
Perphenazine	Hansen et al. (1982)	24–48	26	Yes (C)
Trifluoperazine	Janicak et al. (1989)	10	36	Yes (C)
Butaperazine	Casper et al. (1980)	20–40	24	.32(C)

Note. R = degree of correlation between drug levels in blood and therapeutic response. L = linear correlation; C = curvilinear correlation; Yes = statistically significant correlation, R not calculated; No = correlation not statistically significant, R not calculated.

which patients with the highest and lowest blood levels had worse outcomes than those with intermediate blood levels.

The results of these studies are summarized in Table 1–2. Findings are presented for all studies taken together and for studies of only haloperidol, the most commonly employed drug. Only 17 of all 32 studies (53%) and 9 of the 16 haloperidol studies (56%) revealed statistically significant correlations of drug levels and effects. The observed correlations were usually weak. Curvilinear correlations were sometimes significantly stronger than linear correlations. However, even curvilinear correlations were typically of modest strength, with less than 20% of the variance in outcome explained by differences in blood level.

The meaning of these findings is probably best appreciated by looking at the results of a representative study. In our study of thioridazine (Cohen et al. 1989a), we observed correlations between plasma levels of drug and clinical outcome similar to those seen in the studies in Table 1–1. Figure 1–1 shows our results from this fixed-dose study of thioridazine. The correlation (Spearman) observed between plasma levels of drug and percent improvement in symptoms was $r_s = .19$ $(P = .17)$. As with many of the other

Table 1–2. Summary observations of 32 fixed-dose studies of relationship of plasma concentrations of neuroleptic and clinical response[a]

✦ Total number of patients studied	867 (423 for haloperidol)
✦ Mean number of patients per study	27 (26 for haloperidol)
✦ Mean dose for all studies	16 mg/day
✦ Mean dose in 16 studies of haloperidol	22 mg/day

✦ In 17 of the 32 studies (53%) and 9 of 16 of studies (56%) using haloperidol, a statistically significant correlation between drug level and response was observed.

✦ For the 15 studies testing a linear correlation between drug level and response: mean $R = .21$ (for studies of haloperidol, mean $r = .18$); range $= -.03$ to .62.

✦ For the 16 studies testing a curvilinear correlation between drug level and response: mean $R = .43$ (for studies of haloperidol, mean $r = .43$); range $= .04$ to .69.

✦ In 9 of the 32 studies (28%) an "inverted U-shaped" correlation between drug levels and response was observed. For these studies, the ratio of drug level at the top of the optimal range to drug level at the bottom of the optimal range averaged 4.6 (range $= 2.0$ to 14).

[a]See Table 1–1.

studies noted in Table 1–1, the best fitting curve was an inverted U, which reduced variance by an additional 21%.

What is most striking about the data is the range of improvement seen at every level of drug. Also whereas improvement was, on average, better in the midrange of doses, substantial proportions of patients did well at low, moderate, or high plasma levels of the drug. Thus as suggested by the statistical analyses, plasma level appears to be a relatively weak predictor of

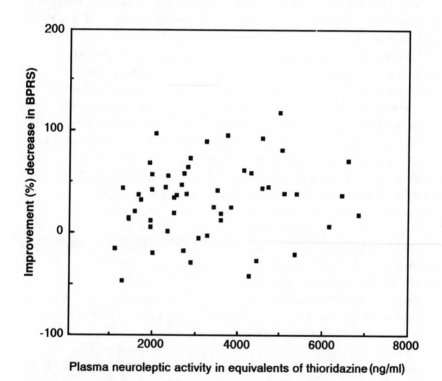

Figure 1–1. Symptomatic improvement versus neuroleptic activity in plasma. Fifty-three patients with an acute exacerbation of psychosis were treated for 2 weeks with a fixed dose of 200 or 400 mg/day of thioridazine. Brief Psychiatric Rating Scale (BPRS; Overall and Gorham 1962) ratings were performed three times weekly, and percent changes in BPRS over 2 weeks were estimated from linear regression. Plasma neuroleptic activity is the mean of three determinations by radioreceptor assay (RRA) in the second week of treatment. Results by RRA and by high-performance liquid chromatography (HPLC) were in high agreement.
Source. From Cohen BM, Lipinski JF, Waternaux C: "A Fixed Dose Study of the Plasma Concentration and Clinical Effects of Thioridazine and Its Major Metabolites." *Psychopharmacology* 97:481–488, 1989. Used with permission.

outcome in the individual case, and it is not evident from visual observation of the data what levels are clearly too high or too low.

It was notable in our study that correlations between plasma levels of drug and side effects were considerably stronger than those between plasma levels of drug and therapeutic effects. Thus the correlation was $r_s = .41$ $(P = .02)$ between plasma level of drug and dry mouth, $r_s = .37$ $(P = .03)$ between plasma level and blurred vision, and $r_s = .21$ $(P = .14)$ between plasma level and sedation. The correlation between total side effects score on a somatic symptoms scale (Cohen et al. 1989a; Kupfer et al. 1989) and plasma level of drug was $r_s = .33$ $(P = .05)$.

It is tempting to speculate that these relatively strong correlations between increasing drug levels and side effects explain the worse clinical outcome observed at higher levels of drug and, therefore, the inverted U-shaped relationship observed overall between drug level and clinical outcome. Supporting this speculation is the observation that most studies, like ours, have found stronger correlations between dose (Baldessarini et al. 1988) or blood level (Cohen et al. 1989a) and side effects than between dose or blood level and therapeutic effects of neuroleptics. Results of a study by Hansen et al. (1982) specifically suggested that the curve relating drug levels to therapeutic effects rose to the left of (i.e., at lower levels than) the curve relating drug levels to side effects. Therapeutic effects fell as blood levels became sufficient to produce noticeable toxic effects. Similar findings were suggested by an analysis of the relationship of dose to therapeutic and side effects averaged over available studies by Baldessarini et al. (1988). Some authors (McEvoy et al. 1986) have suggested that therapeutic effects can be achieved at doses and blood levels of neuroleptics associated with few or minimal side effects.

Taking the data as a whole, there appear to be many patients who improve on relatively low doses (Baldessarini et al. 1988) or at relatively low blood levels of neuroleptics (Cohen et al. 1989a), and there appears on average to be little benefit gained and noticeable risk taken from increasing drug doses beyond moderate levels.

Levels of Neuroleptic at Active Sites in Brain

As noted earlier, the concentration of neuroleptics in blood is primarily studied to provide an approximation of drug in brain. Ultimately, however, investigators and clinicians alike would prefer to know exactly how much drug is present at the active sites in brain. Such information is becoming available through the application of positron-emission tomography (PET) to study occupancy of central monoamine receptors by neuroleptics.

Thus far studies are few, but they have been informative. Notably, maximal occupancy of presumed dopamine, subtype 2 (D_2), receptors appears to be achieved at relatively low plasma levels of haloperidol (6–10 ng/ml; Wolkin et al. 1989) or relatively low doses of chlorpromazine (100 mg/d; Cambon et al. 1987). These findings are consistent with the observation of marked clinical effects of these drugs at low doses and low concentrations in blood (Baldessarini et al. 1988; Cohen et al. 1989a).

Also of interest is a comparison of D_2-receptor occupancy in brain by typical neuroleptic agents and by the atypical but clinically effective antipsychotic neuroleptic clozapine (Table 1–3). During treatment with typical agents, D_2 receptors appear to be fully occupied. However, clozapine does not lead to maximal occupation of D_2 receptors at effective doses and tissue levels. This difference may suggest that the therapeutic effects of clozapine are mediated in part through dopamine receptors other than D_2, such as the newly discovered dopamine, subtype 3 (D_3), 4 (D_4), or 5 (D_5), receptors (Sokoloff et al. 1990; Van Tol et al. 1991; Sunahara et al. 1991), or other monoamine receptors such as the serotonin 5-HT_2 receptor (Meltzer 1989) or α_1-noradrenergic receptors (Cohen and Lipinski 1986a). Alternatively, it may suggest that optimal therapeutic effects do not require full occu-

Table 1–3. Percent of maximal dopamine, subtype 2(D_2), receptor occupancy during neuroleptic treatment of schizophrenia estimated by positron-emission tomography

Drug	n patients	Dose range (mg/day)	Receptor occupancy mean (range)
Chlorpromazine	1	200	80
Thioridazine	1	300	75
Perphenazine	2	8–60	85 (79–88)
Fluphenazine	2	100/2 weeks (decanoate)	98 (96–99)
Haloperidol	8	2–21	89 (75–100)
Clozapine	3	300–600	48 (40–65)

Note. Occupancy of D_2 receptors in brain by neuroleptic drugs during treatment was estimated by displacement of [76]Br-bromospiperone, ^{11}C-methlyspiperone, or ^{11}C-raclopride.
Source. From Cambon et al. 1987; Farde et al. 1988; Coppens et al. 1991; Sedvall 1990.

pancy of D_2 receptors by neuroleptics. The evidence that clozapine is a more effective antipsychotic agent than typical neuroleptics (Kane et al. 1988) suggests that partial occupation of D_2 receptors or modulation of signal transmission through D_2 receptors rather than full blockade may produce a superior therapeutic outcome.

With typical neuroleptics, partial occupation of D_2 receptors probably occurs at rather low doses (again note the studies of Wolkin et al. 1989 and Cambon et al. 1987). We (Cohen et al. 1989a) and others (McEvoy et al. 1986) have suggested studying the use of these low doses of neuroleptics for the treatment of newly admitted patients with psychotic disorders. In addition, analogous to trials of clozapine, we have suggested studies of the effects of dose reduction in patients with chronic psychosis who do not fully remit on traditional dose regimens (Cohen et al. 1989b). Whereas no single approach is ideal for all patients, we have had success with each of these strategies in many of our patients.

When we began our study of the relationship of blood levels to clinical effects of neuroleptics, typical doses of neuroleptics at McLean Hospital were 800 mg of chlorpromazine and 15–20 mg/day of haloperidol for the treatment of acute psychosis. Staff were concerned that treatment with lower doses would not be effective (Cohen and Lipinski 1986b). Since the completion of our study, doses that are the equivalent of 6–10 mg/day of haloperidol and 200–400 mg/day of chlorpromazine are in routine use with many patients receiving even lower doses. The results of a chart-review study (Vuckovic et al. 1990) suggested that these doses are at least as effective as our older higher-dose regimens.

Similarly, we have had frequent success following substantial (50%–75%) reductions of neuroleptic dose in patients with chronic psychotic disorders and disabling residual symptoms (Cohen et al. 1989b). In these patients, we have sometimes observed initial symptomatic worsening lasting several days to a week. However, in most cases, dose reduction has led in the long term to a decrease in negative symptoms and side effects, an increase in patient involvement in structured activities, improved interpersonal relations, and in some cases, a reduction in positive symptoms.

Clinical Usefulness of Obtaining a Blood Level of Neuroleptics

On the average, only modest correlations have been found between blood levels and the clinical effects of neuroleptics in carefully designed and executed studies. These findings suggest that most of the variability in treatment outcome that is observed in the clinical use of neuroleptics is not because of differences in drug metabolism. Instead, the outcome is probably determined more strongly by interindividual differences in responsiveness to drug.

In clinical circumstances, the correlation between drug levels and drug effects is likely to be even weaker than that observed in protocol-based research studies because many factors controlled in research settings cannot be controlled during routine treatment. Thus, the predictive value of a neuroleptic level obtained during treatment is probably low, and little role would seem to exist for the routine measurement of blood levels of neuroleptics in clinical practice.

However, monitoring blood levels of neuroleptics may be useful in special circumstances, for example, in individual patients whose drug absorption or metabolism are expected to change because of illness or the institution of additional medications. Questions of compliance or unusual metabolism can also be addressed through the determination of neuroleptic levels, and obtaining such levels may occasionally be useful in providing confirming evidence to clinical observation that tissue levels of drug are excessively high or low. Of course, caution in interpretation of the results is necessary because for individuals, as for groups, there is little evidence that drug level correlates highly with drug effect.

Drug level studies have been useful in identifying differences in drug metabolism in some patient groups. For example, both blood levels of phenothiazine neuroleptics and side effects are greater in the elderly than in younger adults given equivalent drug dosages (Cohen and Sommer 1988). These results support the common practice of treating older patients with lower doses of phenothiazines. The same may not be true for butyrophenones because metabolic differences between younger and older adults are not consistently observed.

Finally, findings from blood level studies, like those from dose-response studies, have suggested that the optimal range of doses of neuroleptics is lower and narrower than once believed. These findings suggest that the routine practice of increasing the dose of neuroleptic when clinical effect is not optimal may be mistaken. Instead, monitoring side effects, which may indicate that doses are too high, and maintaining lower doses for longer periods of time to allow a full therapeutic effect to emerge may be preferable. Dose reductions in patients who are treatment resistant or those who have clear side effects are also worth more frequent consideration and further study.

References

Alfredsson G, Harnryd C, Wiesel F-A: Effects of sulpiride and chlorpromazine on autistic and positive psychotic symptoms in schizophrenic patients: relationship to drug concentrations. Psychopharmacology (Berl) 85:8–13, 1985

Baldessarini RJ, Cohen BM, Teicher MH: Significance of neuroleptic dose and plasma level in the pharmacologic treatment of psychoses. Arch Gen Psychiatry 45:79–91, 1988

Bigelow LB, Kirch DG, Braun T, et al: Absence of relationship of serum haloperidol concentration and clinical response in chronic schizophrenia: a fixed-dose study. Psychopharmacol Bull 21:66–68, 1985

Bleeker JAC, Dingemans PM, Frohn-de Winter ML, et al: Plasma level and effect of low-dose haloperidol in acute psychosis. Psychopharmacol Bull 20:317–319, 1984

Cambon H, Baron JC, Boulenger JP, et al: In vivo assay for neuroleptic receptor bining in the striatum: positron tomography in humans. Br J Psychiatry 151:824–830, 1987

Campbell A, Herschel M, Sommer B, et al: Circadian changes in the distribution and effects of haloperidol in the rat. Neuropharmacology 21:663–669, 1982

Casper R, Garver DL, Dekirmenjian H, et al: Phenothiazine levels in plasma and red blood cells. Arch Gen Psychiatry 37:301–305, 1980

Clark ML, Kaul PN, Whitfield LR, et al: Chlorpromazine kinetics and clinical response. Psychopharmacol Bull 14:43–45, 1978

Clow A, Theodorou A, Jenner P, et al: Changes in rat striatal dopamine turnover and receptor activity during one year's neuroleptic administration. Eur J Pharmacol 63:135–144, 1980

Cohen BM: The clinical utility of plasma neuroleptic levels, in Guidelines for the Use of Psychotropic Drugs. Edited by Stancer HC. New York, Spectrum Publications, 1984, pp 245–260

Cohen BM: Neuroleptic drugs in the treatment of acute psychosis, in Current Trends in Psychopharmacology. Edited by Casey DE, Christensen AV. Berlin, Germany, Springer-Verlag, 1988, pp 47–61

Cohen BM, Lipinski JF: In vivo potencies of antipsychotic drugs in blocking alpha 1 noradrenergic and dopamine D2 receptors: implications for drug mechanisms of action. Life Sci 39:2571–2580, 1986a

Cohen BM, Lipinski JF: Treatment of acute psychosis with non-neuroleptic agents. Psychosomatics 27 (suppl):7–16, 1986b

Cohen BM, Sommer BR: Metabolism of thioridazine in the elderly. J Clin Psychopharmacol 8:336–339, 1988

Cohen BM, Zubenko GS: In vivo effects of psychotropic agents on the physical properties of cell membranes in the rat brain. Psychopharmacology (Berl) 86:365–368, 1985a

Cohen BM, Zubenko GS: Relevance of genetic variability to clinical psychopharmacology. Psychopharmacol Bull 21:641–650, 1985b

Cohen BM, Herschel M, Aoba A: Neuroleptic, antimuscarinic, and antiadrenergic activity of chlorpromazine, thioridazine, and their metabolites. Psychiatry Res 1:199–208, 1979

Cohen BM, Lipinski JF, Waternaux C: A fixed dose study of the plasma concentration and clinical effects of thioridazine and its major metabolites. Psychopharmacology (Berl) 97:481–488, 1989a

Cohen BM, Benes FB, Baldessarini RJ: Atypical neuroleptics, dose response relationships and treatment-resistant psychosis. Arch Gen Psychiatry 46:381–383, 1989b

Cohen BM, Baldessarini RJ, Campbell A, et al: Persistence of antipsychotic drug effects and tissue levels, in Advances in Schizophrenia Research. Edited by Schulz CR, Tamminga C. New York, Raven, 1991, pp 277–285

Contreras S, Alexander H, Faber R, et al: Neuroleptic radioreceptor activity and clinical outcome in schizophrenia. J Clin Psychopharmacol 7:95–98, 1987

Coppens HJ, Slooff CJ, Paana AMJ, et al: High central D2-dopamine receptor occupancy as assessed with positron emission tomography in medicated but therapy-resistant schizophrenic patients. Biol Psychiatry 29:629–634, 1991

Davis MM, Erickson S, Dekirmenjian H: Plasma levels of antipsychotic drugs and clinical response, in Psychopharmacology: A Generation of Progress. Edited by Lipton MA, DiMascio A, Killiam KF. New York, Raven, 1978, pp 905–916

Dysken MW, Javaid JI, Chang SS, et al: Fluphenazine pharmacokinetics and therapeutic response. Psychopharmacology (Berl) 73:205–210, 1981

Farde L, Wiesel F-A, Halldin C, et al: Central D2-dopamine receptor occupancy in schizophrenic patients treated with antipsychotic drugs. Arch Gen Psychiatry 45:71–76, 1988

Garver DL, Hirschowitz J, Glicksteen GA, et al: Haloperidol plasma and red blood cell levels and clinical antipsychotic response. J Clin Psychopharmacol 4:133–137, 1984

Greenberg JS, Brown WA, Laughren TP, et al: Neuroleptic levels by radioreceptor assay and clinical response during treatment of acute exacerbation of schizophrenia—Some preliminary findings. Psychopharmacol Bull 19:74–78, 1983

Hansen LB, Larsen N-E, Gulmann N: Dose-response relationships of perphenazine in the treatment of acute psychoses. Psychopharmacology (Berl) 78:112–115, 1982

Hitzemann RJ, Garver DL, Mavroidis M, et al: Fluphenazine activity and antipsychotic response. Psychopharmacology (Berl) 90:270–273, 1986

Janicak PG, Javaid JI, Sharma RP, et al: Trifluoperazine plasma levels and clinical response. J Clin Psychopharmacol 9:340–346, 1989

Kane J, Honigfeld G, Singer J, et al: Clozapine for the treatment-resistant schizophrenic. Arch Gen Psychiatry 45:789–796, 1988

Keck PE, Cohen BM, Baldessarini RJ, et al: Time course of antipsychotic effects of neuroleptic drugs. Am J Psychiatry 146:1289–1292 1989

Kirch DG, Bigelow LB, Korpi ER, et al: Serum haloperidol concentration and clinical response in schizophrenia. Schizophr Bull 14:283–289, 1988

Kupfer DJ, Perel JM, Frank E: Adequate treatment with imipramine in continuation treatment. J Clin Psychiatry 50:250–255, 1989

Lader M: Monitoring plasma concentrations of neuroleptics. Pharmakopsych 9:170–177, 1976

Linkowski P, Hubain P, von Frenckell R, et al: Haloperidol plasma levels and clinical response in paranoid schizophrenics. Eur Arch Psychiatry Neurol Sci 234:231–236, 1984

Mavroidis ML, Kanter DR, Hirschowitz J, et al: Clinical response and plasma haloperidol levels in schizophrenia. Psychopharmacology (Berl) 81:354–356, 1983

Mavroidis ML, Kanter DR, Hirschowitz J, et al: Clinical relevance of thiothixene plasma levels. J Clin Psychopharmacol 4:155–157, 1984a

Mavroidis ML, Kanter DR, Hirschowitz J, et al: Therapeutic blood levels of fluphenazine: Plasma or RBC determinations? Psychopharmacol Bull 20:168–170, 1984b

May PRA, Van Putten T: Plasma levels of chlorpromazine in schizophrenia: A critical review of the literature. Arch Gen Psychiatry 35:1081–1087, 1978

May PRA, Van Putten T, Jenden DJ: Chlorpromazine levels and the outcome of treatment in schizophrenic patients. Arch Gen Psychiatry 38:202–207, 1981

McEvoy JP, Stiller RL, Farr R: Plasma haloperidol levels drawn at neuroleptic threshold doses: A pilot study. J Clin Psychopharmacol 6:133–137, 1986

Meltzer HV: Clinical studies on the mechanism of action of clozapine: the dopamine-serotonin hypothesis of schizophrenia. Psychopharmacology (Berl) 99:S18–S27, 1989

Overall JE, Gorham DR: The Brief Psychiatric Rating Scale. Psychol Rep 10:799–812, 1962

Potkin SG, Shen Y, Zhou D, et al: Does a therapeutic window for plasma haloperidol exist? Preliminary Chinese data. Psychopharmacol Bull 21:59–61, 1985

Sakalis G, Curry SH, Mould GP, et al: Physiologic and clinical effects of chlorpromazine and their relationship to plasma level. Clin Pharmacol Ther 13:931–946, 1972

Santos JL, Cabranes JA, Vazquez C, et al: Clinical response and plasma haloperidol levels in chronic and subchronic schizophrenia. Biol Psychiatry 26:381–388, 1989

Sedvall G: PET imaging of dopamine receptors in human basal ganglia: relevance to mental illness. Trends Neurosci 13:302–308, 1990

Shostak M, Perel JM, Stiller RL, et al: Plasma haloperidol and clinical response: A role for reduced haloperidol in antipsychotic activity? J Clin Psychopharmacol 7:394–400, 1987

Smith RC: Plasma haloperidol levels and clinical response. Arch Gen Psychiatry 44:1110–1112, 1987

Smith RC, Baumgartner R, Ravichandran GK, et al: Plasma and red cell levels of thioridazine and clinical response in schizophrenia. Psychiatry Res 12:287–296, 1984

Smith RC, Baumgartner R, Burd A, et al: Haloperidol and thioridazine drug levels and clinical response in schizophrenia: Comparison of gas-liquid chromatography and radioreceptor drug level assays. Psychopharmacol Bull 21:52–58, 1985a

Smith RC, Baumgartner R, Shvartsburd A, et al: Comparative efficacy of red cell and plasma haloperidol as predictors of clinical response in schizophrenia. Psychopharmacology (Berl) 85:449–455, 1985b

Sokoloff P, Giros B, Martres M-P, et al: Molecular cloning and characterization of a novel dopamine receptor (D3) as a target for neuroleptics. Nature 347:146–151, 1990

Sunahara RK, Guan H-C, O'Dowd BF, et al: Cloning of the gene for a human dopamine D5 receptor with higher affinity for dopamine than D1. Nature 350:614–619, 1991

Sunderland T, Cohen BM: Blood to brain distribution of neuroleptics. Psychiatry Res 20:299–305, 1987

Tang SW, Glaister J, Davidson L, et al: Total and free plasma neuroleptic levels in schizophrenic patients. Psychiatry Res 13:285–293, 1984

Van Putten T, May PRA, Marder SR, et al: Plasma levels of thiothixene by radioreceptor assay: Clinical usefulness. Psychopharmacology (Berl) 79:40–44, 1983

Van Putten T, Marder SR, May PRA, et al: Plasma levels of haloperidol and clinical response. Psychopharmacol Bull 21:69–72, 1985

Van Tol HHM, Bunzow JR, Guan H-C, et al: Cloning of the gene for a human dopamine D4 receptor with high affinity for the antipsychotic clozapine. Nature 350:610–614, 1991

Vuckovic A, Cohen BM, Keck P, et al: Neuroleptic dosage regimens in psychotic inpatients: A retrospective comparison. J Clin Psychiatry 51(3):107–109, 1990

Wistedt B, Johanidesz, Omerhodzic M, et al: Plasma haloperidol levels and clinical response in acute schizophrenia. Nord Psykiatr Tidsskr 9–13, 1984

Wode-Helgodt B, Borg S, Fyro B, et al: Clinical effects and drug concentrations in plasma and cerebrospinal fluid in psychotic patients treated with fixed doses of chlorpromazine. Acta Psychiat Scand 58:149–173, 1978

Wolkin A, Brodie JD, Barouche F, et al: Dopamine receptor occupancy and plasma haloperidol levels. Arch Gen Psychiatry 46:482–483, 1989

Neuroleptic Plasma Levels: Methodological Issues, Study Design, and Clinical Applicability

Philip G. Janicak, M.D.
Javaid I. Javaid, Ph.D.
John M. Davis, M.D.

The ideal drug treatment strategy achieves maximum clinical response with a minimum of side effects. In many branches of medicine, monitoring plasma levels rather than drug dose is often the optimal way to reach this goal. In psychiatry, this approach is used for lithium, carbamazepine, valproic acid, and some antidepressants; however, routine plasma level monitoring for most psychoactive drugs remains controversial. In this chapter, we review the clinical utilization of neuroleptic plasma levels by stating the theoretical basis of the blood level–clinical response relationship and review definitions of some commonly used terms in pharmacokinetics. We also consider methodological issues that complicate the interpretation of results of earlier plasma level–clinical response studies; discuss results of neuroleptic plasma level studies in the literature, as well as study designs (models) appropriate to address these issues; and integrate results from existing valid studies to emphasize the clinical applicability of neuroleptic plasma level monitoring.

This research was supported in part by USPHS Grant MH-45465 from the National Institute of Mental Health.

Theoretical Basis for Blood Level Monitoring

If a drug produced immediate pharmacological effects, the monitoring of plasma levels would be unnecessary. For example, one can directly observe the clinical stages of anesthesia and adjust the anesthetic dosage by simply monitoring its effects. On the other hand, if there is a long interval between clinical response and drug administration, weeks may be required to achieve the desired effect. In such situations, if the plasma concentrations required for clinical response are known, doses can be adjusted more rapidly to achieve the proper levels. Such monitoring is also useful when there are large interindividual differences in response to the same dose for the same diagnosis. Because large interindividual variations in plasma levels with the same dose of neuroleptic are now well established, knowledge of the potential therapeutic range for a given agent could provide more precise guidelines for individualized dose adjustment.

Plasma level studies are also important to establish the minimally effective dose. Because the half-life to response with neuroleptics is about 2 weeks, increasing the dose every few days can overrun this lag period, often leading to doses much higher than required. Whereas dose is usually adjusted based on clinical response, knowing the minimally effective level may avoid greater than necessary neuroleptic exposure. Finally, because there is a positive correlation between the plasma level achieved and the dose required, one can estimate the average dose needed to produce a certain concentration. Therefore, monitoring plasma levels can be thought of as a fine tuning of the dose.

The basic assumptions that underlie the relationship between plasma levels and clinical response are

✦ There is an optimum concentration at which maximum pharmacological response will occur.
✦ There is a relationship between the drug concentration in plasma and the site of action.
✦ Pharmacogenetic and environmental factors vary the quantity of neuroleptic that reaches the receptor site in different individuals.

At low concentrations there will be no response, followed by an increased response as levels rise. After the maximum pharmacological response is achieved, further increases in concentration will not enhance response. Thus a plasma level–clinical response relationship may show the typical sigmoidal shape. Furthermore, at higher concentrations, various side effects of a drug may be more prominent, defining the relationship between its plasma level and these side effects. Thus, a composite plot of the clinical benefit versus drug plasma level will result in an inverted U-shaped relationship (Figure 2–1) that defines the range (or "therapeutic window") to achieve optimum benefit. For most drugs, the upper end of the therapeutic window represents toxicity; however, some drugs may actually lose their clinical effectiveness as a result of their action on different receptors at higher concentrations. For a drug that has neither serious toxic effects nor loss of beneficial effects at higher concentrations, the blood level–clinical response relationship will remain sigmoidal.

Pharmacokinetics can be defined as the study of the time course of changes in drug concentration at various sites. It deals with the time-concentration relationship of drug dose, dose form, dose regimen, and route of administration and incorporates information about 1) absorption, 2) distribution, 3) metabolism, and 4) excretion. Application of this information to improve patient care can be referred to as *clinical pharmacokinetics*. Some terms that may be helpful to understanding these issues are briefly defined in Table 2–1.

The pharmacokinetics of several neuroleptics have been adequately reviewed (Balant-Gorgia and Balant 1987). In general, most are well absorbed from the gastrointestinal tract. However, first-pass hepatic metabolism for several compounds can be extensive, resulting in low bioavailability after oral administration. In some cases the bioavailability can be increased 4 to 10 times by administering the drug intramuscularly. For example, we (Schaffer et al. 1982) found that the bioavailability of haloperidol after an oral dose was 38% compared with intramuscular administration.

The bioavailability for chlorpromazine after oral administration was reported to be only 10% of that after intravenous administration (Curry 1981). In addition to a substantial first-pass effect, the systemic clearance of many neuroleptics is high because of a high hepatic extraction ratio; however, most neuroleptics are also distributed extensively (volume of distribution [V_D] around 20 l/kg body weight) because of their highly lipophilic character, and in spite of their high clearance rate, their biological half-life ($t_{1/2}$) is generally about 20 hours. Therefore, the distribution of neuroleptics in various tissues may play an important role in plasma levels of the parent drug.

The primary route of elimination for most neuroleptics is hepatic metabolism and urinary excretion of the unchanged drug may account for less than 1% of the dose administered. Many of the metabolites of various neu-

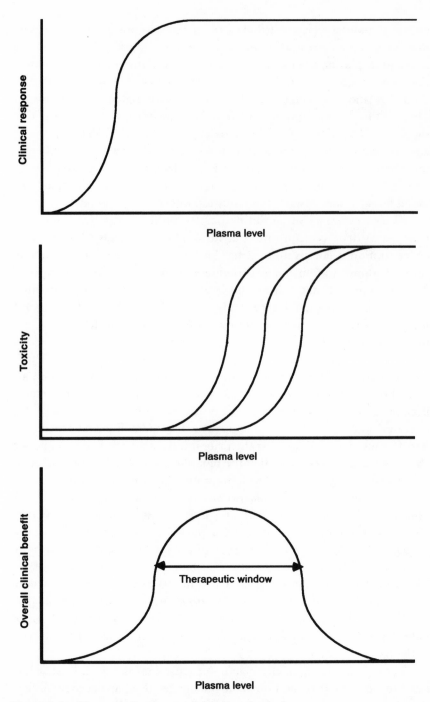

Figure 2–1. Theoretical concept of therapeutic window.

roleptics are also pharmacologically active, thus complicating the relationship between the clinical response and the parent drug blood level. Thus chlorpromazine sulfoxide, 7-hydroxy-chlorpromazine, *N*-didesmethyl-chlorpromazine, and 7-hydroxy-*N*-didesmethylchlorpromazine have been detected in plasma from patients treated with chlorpromazine (Jorgenson 1986). Similarly, reduced haloperidol has been found in plasma (J. I. Javaid, P. G. Janicak, J. M. Davis, unpublished observations, June 1990; Shostak et al. 1987), as well as in postmortem brain tissue of patients who had received haloperidol treatment (Korpi et al. 1984).

Methodological Issues

A number of methodological issues have confounded the interpretation of results, thus minimizing the clinical utility of the plasma level–clinical response relationship (Baldessarini et al. 1988; Dahl 1986; Javaid et al. 1991b). These issues can be grouped as follows: 1) dose strategy, 2) assay method, 3) patient population, and 4) study design.

Table 2–1. Pharmacokinetic factors

Factor	Definition
Absorption	Process by which a drug proceeds from the site of administration to the site of measurement (generally plasma or whole blood)
First-pass effect	Hepatic extraction of orally administered drugs before reaching the systemic circulation
Volume of distribution (V_D)	An indication of drug distribution throughout the body
Steady-state concentration (C_{SS})	The narrow range of drug concentration achieved when the amount administered per unit time equals the amount eliminated per unit time
Clearance (Cl)	A measure of a drug's elimination from the body that relates the plasma concentration to the rate of elimination
Biological half-life ($t_{1/2}$)	Time required for the drug concentration in plasma (or blood) to fall by one-half
Elimination rate constant (K_e)	Percent of drug eliminated per unit of time

Dose Strategy

The most insidious methodological error in plasma level–clinical response studies is the systematic confounding situation of raising the dose when a patient fails to respond. This frequently results in missing the lower end of the therapeutic window because patients are not kept at the lower dose for a sufficient time to document no response. Additionally, because patients respond at a slower rate than the rate of dose increases, some patients who supposedly respond at a higher dose may have actually improved at a lower dose had it been maintained for a longer time. For example, a patient's poor response is caused by a low plasma level. When the clinician increases the dose, the plasma level also rises, and although there may be a response at the higher plasma level frequent repeated dose increases can obscure the low end of a possible therapeutic window or the threshold level for response. In another example, the patient has an adequate plasma level but is refractory. When the dose is increased, the plasma level rises; however, the patient remains nonresponsive at any concentration.

One method of solving confounding situation is to nonrandomly assign a fixed dose based on the patient's clinical condition at admission and then hold it constant throughout the rest of the study. The clinician may initially preassign patients to high, medium, or low doses based on clinical judgment, but this is done before treatment starts and is usually based on the degree of psychosis present. In the absence of a large number of well-designed studies, this method is less rigorous but usable in the interpretation of dose-response studies.

A more effective way to define the plasma level–clinical response relationship is to use a constant- (or fixed-)dose design, regardless of severity of psychosis. It can be a single fixed dose or random assignment to several different fixed doses (perhaps low, medium, and high) to investigate the low and high end of a potential therapeutic window. When data from several fixed-dose studies indicate a possible therapeutic range for a specific drug, prospectively targeting patients to various plasma levels can also be a meaningful method. In this design, patients are maintained in a predetermined fixed plasma level range during the treatment period. This strategy is further discussed under the section on haloperidol studies.

Assay Methods

Several analytical techniques have been used over the years for the quantitation of neuroleptics (Cimbura 1972; Cohen et al. 1980; Dhar and Kutt

1984; Heyes and Salmon 1978; Javaid et al. 1981, 1982a; Jemal et al. 1987; Szczepanik-VanLeeuwen 1985; White et al. 1976; Wiles and Franklin 1979; Wurzburger et al. 1981). Presently, gas-liquid chromatography (GLC) and high-pressure liquid chromatography (HPLC) methods are the most commonly used for such analyses.

Analytical techniques can broadly be divided into chemical or biological assays. Chemical methods primarily use physicochemical characteristics of a drug in conjunction with some instrumentation and are generally individualized for each compound or group of similar compounds. In contrast, biological methods are based on some biological activity of the drug. In general, they do not quantitate the specific drug concentration but rather the activity of the drug is transformed into a concentration equivalent. As a result, these methods cannot distinguish between compounds that have similar biological activities. This problem is highlighted by studies involving neuroleptics because many laboratories have used radioreceptor assays (RRAs) for drug measurements. We have shown that in the same plasma sample, chemical assay and RRA resulted in substantially different levels for various neuroleptics (Javaid et al. 1980) (Table 2–2). Since RRA also measures pharmacologically active metabolites, this outcome was not surprising. A brief description of the principles of these methods along with their utility is given in Table 2–3.

In earlier studies the method of blood collection and sample handling before analysis could also have resulted in variable plasma level measurements. For example, it has been reported that during blood collection of tricyclic antidepressants (Cochran et al. 1978) and phenothiazine neuroleptics (Javaid et al. 1980) contact with rubber stoppers for extended periods of time could result in spuriously low plasma levels.

Table 2–2. Antipsychotic levels by gas-liquid chromatography (GLC) and radioreceptor assays (RRA)

Drug	n	GLC (ng/ml)	RRA (ng/ml)
Haloperidol	20	7.2	10.1
Butaperazine	10	152.0	201.0
Fluphenazine	20	0.97	7.1
Trifluoperazine	35	0.7	5.7

Note. The same plasma sample was analyzed by both methods.
Source. Adapted from Javaid et al. (1982b).

Table 2–3. Various techniques used for the analysis of antipsychotics

Method	Principle	Comments
Chemical assays		
Spectrometric	Drug is extracted into organic solvent and subsequently measured by colorimetric reaction or fluorescence.	At therapeutic concentrations, sensitivity—fair to poor for potent antipsychotics; specificity—poor to fair; rarely used at present.
GLC	Compounds are separated between moving gas phase and stationary liquid phase and detected by different detectors; the method is individualized for each compound or a group of similar compounds after extraction.	The use of specific detectors, such as electron capture (ECD) and nitrogen/phosphorus (NPD), gives good-to-excellent sensitivity and specificity; commonly used in many laboratories for routine measurements.
HPLC	Compounds are separated between moving liquid phase and a stationary phase and detected by different detectors; the method is individualized for each compound or a group of similar compounds after extraction.	The use of special detectors, such as fluorescence or electrochemical detectors, results in good-to-excellent sensitivity and specificity; commonly used in many laboratories for routine measurements.
GC–MS	After extraction, the compounds are separated by GC and fragmented by MS; each compound gives specific mass fragments.	Very specific, with good-to-excellent sensitivity; not economical for routine analysis; generally used to establish specificities for other techniques.

Biological assays

RRA

Radiolabeled drug bound to receptors can be displaced by unlabeled compounds with similar binding characteristics; the plasma can be used without extraction.

This method measures the inhibitory activity of the sample; although simple, with fair sensitivity, the method has poor specificity; some laboratories use in clinical studies

RIA

Antibodies are prepared against the drug linked to a protein; the displacement by the sample of radiolabeled drug from antibody-antigen complex is determined; the sample can be used without extraction.

The method is sensitive and simple; however, the specificity is poor to fair and depends on the cross-reactivity of structurally related compounds; generally restricted to the laboratories that have specific antibodies because currently they are not commercially available.

Note. GLC = gas-liquid chromatography; HPLC = high-pressure liquid chromatography; GC–MS = gas chromatography-mass spectrometry; RRA = radioreceptor assay; RIA = radioimmunoassay.
Source. Adapted from Javaid et al. (1991b).

Patient Population

Patient population issues include: the inclusion of refractory patients; a nonhomogeneous patient sample; patient noncompliance, particularly in outpatient studies; and small patient sample size. More recent studies have distinguished between neuroleptic-responsive versus refractory patients, utilized more rigorous criteria to assure homogeneity in diagnosis, and increased the sample size to allow for adequate analysis.

Study Design

Important issues relating to study design include: inadequate evaluation of clinical response; concurrent, multiple drug treatments; too brief an observation period; and variable time of blood sampling. As noted earlier, the interpretation of plasma level versus clinical response data even in well-designed studies is further complicated by the presence of many active metabolites formed by biotransformation, the major route of elimination for neuroleptics.

Neuroleptic Plasma Levels

Neuroleptics are a chemically diverse group effective in ameliorating various psychotic symptoms. However, they can also induce significant adverse effects such as the neuroleptic malignant syndrome and various tardive syndromes (e.g., tardive dyskinesia and dystonia). Most important, a significant percentage of patients fail to adequately respond. Whereas large interindividual variability in the steady-state plasma concentrations among patients treated with similar doses of a given neuroleptic is well established, the existence of a critical range of plasma concentration for clinical response or significant side effects remains controversial. However, there is a body of data indicating a possible relationship between neuroleptic plasma concentrations and clinical response.

Chlorpromazine

Curry and colleagues (Curry 1968; Curry et al. 1970a, 1970b) found a wide range of effective plasma drug levels in schizophrenic patients treated with comparable doses of chlorpromazine. They established that an upward or downward shift of 50% in dosage usually produced side effects or a return of psychotic symptoms, respectively. In one patient who had not responded to 1,900 mg daily po chlorpromazine, a reduction in the dose by one-third not only resulted in a corresponding reduction in the plasma level but also a satisfactory clinical response. Wode-Helgodt et al. (1978) studied chlorpromazine concentrations in 44 schizophrenic patients treated with different doses in a constant-dose design. They found a positive correlation between plasma levels and clinical response, suggesting a lower threshold level of 40 ng/ml. By contrast, May et al. (1981), treated 48 psychotic patients with fixed doses of chlorpromazine (6.6 mg/kg body weight per day) and found no relationship between plasma levels and response.

Butaperazine

Garver et al. (1977) reported that in 10 patients treated with butaperazine, plasma levels below 40 ng/ml showed no change in clinical symptomatology, in contrast to patients with plasma levels between 40 ng/ml and 265 ng/ml who showed different degrees of improvement. Smith et al. (1979) studied blood levels of butaperazine in patients with chronic schizophrenia who did not respond as compared with those who had generally shown a better clinical response and found that nonresponsive patients had two to seven times lower levels of plasma and red blood cell butaperazine concentrations than those who responded. This study also implied that low blood levels of neuroleptics may be an important factor in the poor clinical response of some patients with chronic schizophrenia.

Fluphenazine

Several groups have investigated fluphenazine plasma levels in patients receiving either the oral or the intramuscular decanoate form of fluphenazine. Clinical response as a function of mean steady-state fluphenazine levels after oral administration suggested an upper end of the therapeutic window based on three patients who responded poorly and had mean steady-state values above 2.8 ng/ml (Dysken et al. 1981). Furthermore, a lower end was suggested by two nonresponsive patients and one partially responsive patient with levels below 0.2 ng/ml.

More recently, Van Putten et al. (1991) noted that higher fluphenazine levels (up to 4.23 ng/ml) were significantly associated ($P < .02$) with a higher rate of improvement; however, 90% of patients (65 of 72) experienced disabling side effects at a plasma fluphenazine level of 2.7 ng/ml. Marder et al. (1990) found significant relationships ($P < .04$ and $P < .005$) between fluphenazine plasma levels and psychotic exacerbations after 6 or

9 months of maintenance therapy as part of a 2-year double-blind comparison of 5 mg versus 25 mg of fluphenazine decanoate in 39 schizophrenic patients. Thus, those patients with levels less than 0.5 ng/ml did much worse than those with levels above 1.0 ng/ml.

Perphenazine

Hansen et al. (1982) assigned patients to oral perphenazine doses based on clinical condition with an average dosage of 30.5 mg/day (range: 12–48 mg/day). They found that levels of 2 nmol/l or below were usually ineffective (i.e., only 1 out of 7 patients improved), whereas levels over 2 nmol/l were very effective (i.e., 19 out of 19 patients improved). Thus there appeared to be a threshold effect, with lower plasma levels producing a poor response.

Thiothixene

Yesavage et al. (1983) treated 48 acute schizophrenic patients with 80 mg/day of thiothixene, measuring serum and red blood cell concentrations 2 hours after the morning dose. Serum levels ranged from 3 to 45 ng/ml, with a linear relation between clinical response during the first week of treatment and serum levels ($r = .5$), as well as for red blood cell levels ($r = .64$). By contrast, Mavroidis et al. (1984) reported a curvilinear relationship between thiothixene plasma levels and clinical response. Levels ranging between 2.0 and 15 ng/ml, measured 10 to 12 hours after the dose, were associated with clinical improvement; however, of 19 patients, only 1 had plasma levels greater than 15 ng/ml.

Trifluoperazine

Recently, our group (Janicak et al. 1989) reported on a potential therapeutic window with the commonly used phenothiazine, trifluoperazine. We treated an acutely psychotic group of patients ($N = 36$) with a relatively low, fixed dose (5 mg bid) for 2 weeks and correlated clinical improvement with plasma levels at the end of this treatment phase. As with previous neuroleptic studies, there was a wide interindividual difference in steady-state levels (i.e., range = 0.20–3.50 ng/ml or an 18-fold difference). We also found evidence for a lower therapeutic threshold, around 1 ng/ml, and a suggestion of an upper end around 2.3 ng/ml (Table 2–4). Although trifluoperazine is known to have active metabolites in plasma, it is unknown whether they pass the blood-brain barrier, and because we only measured the parent compound, we cannot comment on their potential impact. Although there was some heterogeneity in the diagnostic categories (i.e., 30 patients were diagnosed as having schizophrenia, 5 as having schizoaffective disease, and 1 as having unspecified functional psychosis), the design was such that a drug response was fully expected because all patients had experienced a recent, florid, clearly ratable, psychotic exacerbation (i.e., delusions and/or hallucinations) requiring acute hospitalization. All patients improved sufficiently during the index admission (average hospital stay approximately 2 months) to be discharged to outpatient care. Further, when the results were analyzed using only those 30 patients diagnosed as having schizophrenia, the results were virtually identical.

Based on our review of neuroleptic dose-response studies, 9–15 mg of trifluoperazine would be roughly equivalent to 300 mg of chlorpromazine and should fall near the lower part of the linear portion of the dose-response curve. Indeed, with a 10-mg dose, we appear to have found a lower end (1 ng/ml plasma) to a postulated therapeutic window in our patient sample that is consistent with our previous predicted dose-response calculations. Furthermore, there were tentative data defining a potential upper end (i.e., 2.3 ng/ml plasma) of the therapeutic window for this drug.

Haloperidol

Haloperidol is the most commonly prescribed neuroleptic and unlike most others it has only one pharmacologically active metabolite (i.e., reduced

Table 2–4. Average change scores on the BPRS and GAS by trifluoperazine plasma level category

| Plasma level category | n | Mean change scores | |
		BPRS	GAS
Low (< 1 ng/ml)	19	– 0.74 (± 8.7)	4.2 (± 11.4)
Medium (> 1 ng/ml; < 2.3 ng/ml)	12	14.7 (± 11.4)	16.0 (± 12.3)
High (> 2.3 ng/ml)	5	1.4 (± 5.5)	2.4 (± 8.1)

Note. BPRS = Brief Psychiatric Rating Scale (Overall and Gorham 1962); GAS = Global Assessment Scale (Spitzer et al. 1973).

haloperidol). Although numerous researchers have examined the relationship between haloperidol steady-state plasma levels and clinical response, they have used varied methodologies in terms of patient selection, symptom profile, diagnostic criteria, assay techniques, and the use of variable- or fixed-dose schedules. Therefore, the results of these studies are difficult to interpret collectively. As with other neuroleptics, the results with the fixed-dose studies of haloperidol have also been conflicting, although at least six studies (Garver et al. 1984; Mavroidis et al. 1983; Potkin et al. 1985; Santos et al. 1989; Smith et al. 1984; Van Putten et al. 1985, 1988) have demonstrated a curvilinear relationship (i.e., therapeutic window) between plasma levels and clinical response. Although optimal levels differed slightly among these studies, we found the mean low end was 4.7 ng/ml (±2.1) and the high end was 17.1 ng/ml (±5.4) (Table 2–5).

Mavroidis et al. (1983) studied 14 DSM-III (American Psychiatric Association 1980) schizophrenic patients for 2 weeks. After a 2-day washout, patients were randomly assigned to fixed dosages of 6, 12, or 24 mg/day for 14 days. Patients were rated with the New Haven Schizophrenic Index (NHSI; Astrachan et al. 1972), and plasma haloperidol was measured by

Table 2–5. Fixed-dose studies finding a curvilinear relationship between haloperidol plasma levels and clinical response

Study	Assay method	Therapeutic range (ng/ml)	Scale	Duration (weeks)
Mavroidis et al. (1983) and Garver et al. (1984)	GLC	3–11	NHSI	2
Smith et al. (1984)	GLC (RRA)	7–17	BPRS[a]	3.5
Potkin et al. (1985)	RIA	4–26 (or 1–22)	CGI	6
Van Putten et al. (1985)	RIA	5–16	BPRS	1
Van Putten et al. (1988)	RIA	2–12	BPRS[a]	4
Santos et al. (1989)	RIA	12–35.5 (7.4–24.9 in subchronic group)	BPRS[b]	3

Note. GLC = gas-liquid chromatography; RRA = radioreceptor assay; NHSI = New Haven Schizophrenic Index (Astrachan et al. 1972); BPRS = Brief Psychiatric Rating Scale (Overall and Gorham 1962); CGI = Clinical Global Impression Scale (National Institute of Mental Health 1985).
[a]Psychosis factor.
[b]Total score.

GLC. This study suggested that a curvilinear relationship existed between haloperidol plasma levels and NHSI ratings (i.e., at least a 40% improvement) with a therapeutic window between 4.2–11 ng/ml. In a study of red blood cell and plasma haloperidol levels (also measured by GLC) in the same patient population, Garver et al. (1984) found evidence for a plasma therapeutic range (3–11 ng/ml) by day 14 of treatment using three fixed dosages (i.e., 6, 12, or 24 mg/day). Seventeen patients who met DSM-III criteria for schizophrenia in acute exacerbation were assessed for changes in baseline pathology with the serial modified NHSI. Those whose levels were within this range ($n = 6$) showed a significantly better response than those with levels outside it ($n = 8$, $P < .01$).

Smith et al. (1984) studied 27 schizophrenic or schizoaffective patients (as diagnosed by the Research Diagnostic Criteria [RDC; Spitzer et al. 1978]) over 24 days. They excluded patients with a history of nonresponse to neuroleptics, long inpatient hospitalizations, or lack of predominance of positive symptoms from the study. Patients were kept drug free from 1 to 3 weeks and then randomly assigned to 10 or 25 mg/day of haloperidol. Blood was drawn 11.5 hours after the last dose and plasma levels were measured by both GLC and RRA. They reported a curvilinear relationship between the GLC-measured plasma levels and the Brief Psychiatric Rating Scale (BPRS; Overall and Gorham 1962) psychosis factor, with maximum efficacy related to plasma levels between 7–17 ng/ml. Even though a subsequent letter by Smith (1987) reported an inability to replicate their original results, when the data were combined (i.e., the old and new samples, excluding the presumed chronic "nonresponders"), a significant relationship persisted.

Potkin et al. (1985) studied 43 schizophrenic and schizophreniform patients diagnosed by DSM-III criteria (17 to 45 years old) with an illness duration less than 5 years. Patients were drug free for 1 week and randomly assigned to a fixed-dose schedule of either 0.4 or 0.15 mg/kg body weight of haloperidol for 45 days. The Clinical Global Impression (CGI) Scale (National Institute of Mental Health 1985) and the BPRS were used on days 7, 14, 28, and 42. Plasma levels were obtained 12 hours after the last dose and were measured by radioimmunoassay (RIA). This study again suggested a curvilinear relationship between blood levels and CGI and BPRS ratings, with a therapeutic window between 4.0–26.0 ng/ml.

Van Putten et al. (1985) studied 47 schizophrenic patients who were drug free for up to 3 weeks and then randomly assigned to fixed dosages of 5, 10, or 20 mg/day of haloperidol. After 4 weeks the dose for nonresponsive patients was increased up to 30 mg/day for another 4 weeks. Patients were evaluated with the BPRS, Nurses' Observation Scale for Inpatient Evaluation (NOSIE; Honigfeld and Klett 1965), and CGI rating scales. Blood was drawn 12 hours after the last dose and haloperidol measured by RIA. They reported a curvilinear relationship between the BPRS and CGI scales and plasma levels only during the first week of treatment, with a therapeutic range of 5–16 ng/ml, and also noted that the daily dose positively correlated with plasma levels. A second study by Van Putten et al. (1988) included 76 male schizophrenic patients, used an RIA assay, and found a curvilinear relationship (i.e., 2–12 ng/ml) between haloperidol plasma levels and the BPRS psychosis factor after 4 weeks of treatment.

Santos et al. (1989) treated 30 schizophrenic patients with three randomly assigned doses of haloperidol (15, 20, and 30 mg/day) for 21 days, after at least 10 days washout from oral medications and 4 months from depot neuroleptics. Ten patients each were assigned to one of the three fixed-dose groups and plasma levels were determined on treatment days 4, 7, 14, and 21 with RIA. The authors found evidence for an inverted U-shaped relationship between the percent improvement from baseline on the total BPRS and the steady-state concentration (C_{SS}) of haloperidol, with an overall effective concentration range of 12.0 to 35.5 ng/ml. When patients' illnesses were classified as subchronic or chronic, however, the therapeutic ranges were 7.4 to 24.9 ng/ml and 14.8 to 38.5 ng/ml, respectively. Santos et al. postulated that, possibly because of the development of tolerance in the dopamine system(s), the effective concentration interval may vary with chronicity of illness.

Two other studies with alternate methodologies had similar findings. Magliozzi et al. (1981) reported a fixed-dose study on 17 patients (16 outpatients) over a period of 3–12 weeks. The fixed dosages ranged from 2 to 120 mg/day with plasma levels ranging from undetectable to 96 ng/ml. Of the 17 individuals, 2 had their doses changed during the study. Magliozzi used an "index of improvement" to determine response and showed that improvement was significantly greater ($P < .001$) for patients who had a mean haloperidol serum concentration between 8 and 18 ng/ml. Davis et al. (1985) conducted a 3-week fixed-dose study in 25 acutely decompensated schizophrenic patients. This was a comparison study of high-dose haloperidol (60 mg/day im for 5 days, followed by 45, 30, and 20 mg/day po for 2, 2, and 3 days, respectively, and then 15 mg/day po for the final week of the study) versus a standard-dose group (15 mg/day po for 3 weeks). They found that 43% of the patients who responded had plasma levels between 5 and 21 ng/ml, in contrast to only 10% of the patients who did not respond.

A number of studies have shown a linear relationship or no correlation at all between plasma haloperidol and clinical response. Volavka and Cooper (1987) reviewed seven haloperidol fixed-dose studies and found that two demonstrated a linear relationship and five demonstrated no relationship. The studies with a linear relationship had used low doses (6 mg/day and 0.2 mg/kg body weight per day, respectively); therefore, it may be that they were reaching only the lower limits of a possible therapeutic window. Of the five studies that showed no relationship at all, two used chronically ill patients and one used a heterogeneous group with psychotic disorders. Perry et al. (1988) reviewed five studies that included only schizophrenic patients who were on fixed-dose schedules, were treated for 2 or more weeks, and demonstrated at least a 30% improvement on the BPRS. Using a logistic regression analysis, they felt that these studies together demonstrated a linear rather than a curvilinear relationship between haloperidol plasma levels and clinical response. And finally, Volavka et al. (1992) failed to find evidence for a therapeutic window after randomly assigning 176 schizophrenic or schizoaffective patients to one of three haloperidol plasma levels (i.e., 2–13; 13.1–24; or 24.1–35 ng/ml) for 6 weeks. Patients who did not improve were then reassigned to another level for an additional 6 weeks. Interpretation of Volavka et al.'s results, however, may be complicated by too high a level for the low and middle ranges and the period of time to titrate to the middle and high haloperidol plasma levels (i.e., approximately 2 weeks).

In summary, results from a number of plasma level studies have indicated a possible curvilinear (inverted U-shaped) or linear relationship with clinical response for such neuroleptics as chlorpromazine (Wode-Helgodt et al. 1978), butaperazine (Casper et al. 1984; Garver et al. 1977), fluphenazine (Chang et al. 1985; Dysken et al. 1981), perphenazine (Hansen and Larsen 1985), thiothixene (Mavroidis et al. 1984), trifluoperazine (Janicak et al. 1989), and haloperidol (Davis et al. 1985; Garver et al. 1984; Mavroidis and Garver 1985; Potkin et al. 1985; Smith et al. 1984; Van Putten et al. 1985); although not all studies find such relationships. What is needed are prospective studies targeting large numbers of acutely ill patients to certain plasma levels to test the hypothesis of a therapeutic threshold or range.

Preliminary Results from a Targeted Plasma-Level Study Design

Thus far, the most valid experimental design for examining the relationship between blood level and clinical response has used fixed doses and analyzed the relationship retrospectively. However, in many of these studies, the number of patients who did not respond at higher plasma levels was very small. Furthermore, because the data were analyzed after the completion of the study, we do not know if these patients would have responded by reducing the plasma levels with dose reduction. There are also statistical problems with a post hoc assignment to a given plasma level category using data from a single study. However, because the plasma level–clinical response relationship may be nonlinear, it is helpful to characterize this relationship with the initial data so that subsequent validation studies can be conducted. To confirm such a categorization one could pool data from several studies to achieve an adequate sample size that would clearly define the optimal cutoff point for a lower end, and possibly for an upper end as well, and then use these data to design a targeted plasma level study.

Because such data are available for haloperidol, we, as well as others (Volavka et al. 1992), are presently conducting targeted plasma level studies to prospectively test the hypothesis of a curvilinear relationship with haloperidol. In our study design, patients hospitalized with an acute exacerbation of their psychosis were initially randomly assigned in a double-blind design to one of three empirical dosages (2, 5, or 10 mg bid) to achieve a targeted haloperidol C_{SS} range of < 5 ng/ml (low group), 6–18 ng/ml (middle group), or ≥ 25 ng/ml (high group). If a patient did not achieve the assigned range after 5 days, the dose was adjusted using the formula

$$D_2 = D_1 \cdot C_{SS2}/C_{SS1}$$

in which D_1 is the original dose, D_2 is the new dose required for the targeted C_{SS2}, and C_{SS1} is the observed steady-state concentration with the original dose.

As part of this study we developed a formula to more rapidly achieve the desired haloperidol C_{SS}. For this purpose the first 28 patients, before receiving the initial assigned dose for achieving their targeted level, received a 15-mg test dosage (po) of haloperidol and blood samples were drawn 24 and 48 hours after the dose. Data analysis indicated a strong linear relationship between the targeted log C_{SS} achieved and the dose required when the 24-hour log plasma level was included in a linear regression model ($r = .933$) (Javaid et al. 1991a).

Having developed this formula, we are now prospectively testing its validity to determine the dose required to achieve the desired haloperidol C_{SS}. Thus far, this method has decreased the time required to achieve the targeted plasma level from 7.2 (± 4.3) to 4.8 (± 2.3) days (Table 2–6).

Once the targeted C_{SS} range is achieved, a patient is maintained on the same dose for 2 weeks. If there is a 30% or greater improvement from the baseline BPRS score, patients are classified as "responders" and remain in their assigned plasma level range group for 2 more weeks. Half of the initial "nonresponders" in the low and high groups are reassigned to the middle group, and half of the middle-level initial "nonresponders" are assigned to the high group to ascertain whether they then convert to a "responder" status. The other half of the patients who did not respond remain in their originally assigned group to control for the effect of time on treatment response. We hope that the results of such a prospective study will unequivocally establish the existence of a plasma level–clinical response relationship for haloperidol, if indeed it exists.

Thus far, 53 patients have entered the study, following an average in-hospital washout of 12.1 (±5.7) days. Preliminary results are described in Tables 2–7, 2–8, and 2–9 and in Figure 2–1. Forty-two have successfully completed at least treatment phase A, with the mean plasma haloperidol C_{SS} achieved for the three groups as follows:

◆ Low ($n = 18$) = 2.07 ng/ml; range = 0.2 to 4.9 ng/ml
◆ Middle ($n = 11$) = 12.7 ng/ml; range = 6.8 to – 17.5 ng/ml
◆ High ($n = 13$) = 44.4 ng/ml; range = 25.0 to – 77.8 ng/ml

In the low group, five initial "nonresponders" were then randomly reassigned to the middle group, and two of these converted to "responders" during treatment phase B (i.e., 40%). By comparison, one of five (20%) initial "nonresponders" assigned to remain in the low group converted to a "responder". Finally, one of six (17%) initial "responders" randomly assigned to remain in the low group during treatment phase B worsened. Because of administrative issues, patient uncooperativeness, or improvement to the point of discharge, we have minimal data for the middle group

Table 2–6. Number of days required to achieve the targeted haloperidol plasma level using two different dosing models

Empirically derived model ($n = 37$)	Formula derived model ($n = 32$)
7.2 (±4.3) days	4.8 (±2.3) days
Low = 15 (41%)	Low = 4 (41%)
Middle = 11 (35%)	Middle = 2 (25%)
High = 9 (24%)	High = 6 (34%)

Table 2–7. Preliminary data of targeted haloperidol study: low group

Patient	Sex	Age (years)	Diagnosis	Days completed	Response A	mg/day	Level	Response B	mg/day	Level
01	M	35	S	35	Yes	4	1.3	Yes	4	2.7
03[a]	M	27	S	41	No	4	3.2	Yes	20	16.9
08	F	34	SA-A	29	No	4	0.6	Yes	10	2.1
09	M	35	S	36	Yes	4	2.4	Yes	4	1.7
11	F	34	S	28	No	4	0.75	No	10	2.1
14	F	25	S	35	Yes	4	2	No	4	2.2
16	M	22	S	30	Yes	4	0.79	Yes	4	0.65
20[a]	M	32	S	46	No	4	2.6	No	16	11.9
25	F	34	S	30	No	4	1.4	No	4	1.6
31	F	30	S	37	No	4	3.1	No	4	1.9
32	F	22	S	35	Yes	4	1.0	Yes	4	1.9
34	F	44	S	14	No	4	3.5	—	—	—
36	F	28	S	12	—	—	—	—	—	—
38	F	32	SA-A	35	Yes	4	2.1	Yes	4	3.3
40[a]	F	32	SA-S	35	No	4	4.9	No	4	8.9
42	M	29	S	29	No	4	0.2	—	—	—
46	M	43	S	35	No	8	2.6	No	8	2.5
49[a]	M	29	S	44	No	2	1.98	Yes	18	10.9
53[a]	M	33	SA-A	50	No	4	3.0	No	20	14.0
55	M	30	S	38	No	4	4.6	No	4	1.0

Note. Four patients dropped out from the low group; two patients refused to cooperate, and two dropped out because of clinical deterioration. S = schizophrenia; SA-A = schizoaffective, mainly affective; SA-S = schizoaffective, mainly schizophrenic.
[a]Patient who did not respond in treatment phase A, who was randomly reassigned to the middle plasma level in treatment phase B.

Table 2–8. Preliminary data of targeted haloperidol study: middle group

Patient	Sex	Age (years)	Diagnosis	Days completed	Response A	mg/day	Level	Response B	mg/day	Level
02	M	18	SA-S	39	No	20	12.7	No	20	10.9
04	M	42	SA-S	25	Yes	15	14.2	—	—	—
05	F	52	S	28	Yes	22	16.9	—	—	—
12	F	34	S	12	—	—	—	—	—	—
15	F	27	S	48	No	60	16.2	No	60	14
17	F	29	S	6	—	—	—	—	—	—
18	F	35	S	27	—	—	—	—	—	—
19	M	34	S	12	Yes	10	8.5	—	—	—
21	F	32	S	43	No	30	15.5	Yes	30	12.7
22	F	31	S	35	No	8	11.8	Yes	8	11.8
23	F	32	SA-S	15	—	—	—	—	—	—
24	M	42	S	30	No	14	10.4	—	—	—
27	F	49	S	20	—	—	—	—	—	—
28	M	30	S	21	—	—	—	—	—	—
35	M	27	SA-S	35	Yes	16	9.0	No	16	10.0
39	M	30	S	12	—	—	—	—	—	—
47	M	21	SA-S	15	No	28	17.5	—	—	—
50	M	28	SA-S	21	No	22	6.8	—	—	—

Note. Thirteen patients dropped out from the middle group—four patients because of side effects; two patients because of clinical deterioration; three patients because of an inability to achieve a proper level; and four patients dropped out at their request. S = schizophrenia; SA-S = schizoaffective, mainly schizophrenic.

Table 2–9. Preliminary data of targeted haloperidol study: high group

Patient	Sex	Age (years)	Diagnosis	Days completed	Response A	mg/day	Level	Response B	mg/day	Level
06	M	37	S	41	Yes	48	39.6	No	48	61.05
07	F	44	S	43	Yes	70	70.2	Yes	70	40.6
10[a]	M	21	S	56	No	70	25.0	Yes	34	19.0
13	M	27	S	7	—	—	—	—	—	—
26[a]	M	38	S	49	No	60	40.0	Yes	50	22.4
29	F	49	S	20	—	—	—	—	—	—
30	F	33	SA-A	28	No	30	34.4	No	60	69.0
33	F	18	SA-S	41	Yes	60	71.8	—	—	—
37	F	40	SA-A	28	No	50	35.5	—	—	—
41	F	28	SA-S	13	No	30	43.3	Yes	16	11.6
43[a]	F	29	SA-O	45	No	60	45.6	—	—	—
44	F	19	S	14	—	—	—	—	—	—
45	F	27	SA-S	36	Yes	30	63.0	Yes	30	50.7
48	M	19	S	34	Yes	38	45.9	No	38	20.6
51	M	24	SA-S	21	Yes	44	27.8	—	—	—
52	M	26	S	27	No	60	35.1	—	—	—
54	M	33	S	7	—	—	—	—	—	—
56	F	29	S	—	Yes	30	27.5	—	30	—
58[a]	F	31	—	—	No	50	23.6	—	20	—

Note. Nine patients dropped out from the high group: two patients dropped out because of clinical deterioration; five dropped out at their request; one was uncooperative; and one had significant hypotension. S = schizophrenia; SA-A = schizoaffective, mainly affective; SA-S = schizoaffective, mainly schizophrenic; SA-O = schizoaffective, mainly other.
[a]Patient who did not respond in treatment phase A, who was randomly reassigned to the middle plamsa level in treatment phase B.

at this juncture and can only comment that two of four (50%) of the initial "nonresponders" assigned to remain in the middle group converted to "responders" during phase B. In the initial high group, three of four (75%) "nonresponders" randomly reassigned to the middle group converted to "responders". By contrast, three of five (60%) initial "responders" in the high group worsened in treatment phase B.

Conclusions

A substantial number of studies show large differences in plasma levels among patients treated with the same doses of a neuroleptic. This provides one rationale for the clinician to adjust the dose based on blood levels of the drug to achieve the optimal clinical effect. However, the putative therapeutic ranges must be established for each individual drug. It is also necessary for various analytical laboratories to agree on exact limits. Thus a large body of information is required before even a rough approximation of the therapeutic range can be determined.

Unlike sodium, plasma levels of neuroleptics differ widely among individuals because of differences in their rates of metabolism. Therefore, the clinician must adjust each patient's dosage to achieve maximum benefit with minimal side effects. We believe the best way to understand plasma levels is not through arbitrarily selected numbers defining the upper or lower limits of the therapeutic window, but by assessing the clinical utility of a given plasma level in the context of the published data from methodologically valid studies.

Routine plasma level monitoring for most of the neuroleptics is experimental at this point. However, plasma level monitoring can be useful in conjunction with clinical assessment for the following situations:

- ✦ To determine patient compliance
- ✦ To establish adequacy of the pharmacotherapy in patients who do not respond to treatment
- ✦ To maximize the clinical response where the drug plasma level–clinical response relationship is elucidated
- ✦ To help define the dose-response relationship
- ✦ To avoid toxicity because of unnecessarily high plasma levels
- ✦ In patients with other medical disorders and/or on concurrent medical drugs
- ✦ As a safeguard for the clinician in potential medical-legal situations

References

American Psychiatric Association: Diagnostic and Statistical Manual of Mental Disorders, 3rd Edition. Washington, DC, American Psychiatric Association, 1980

Astrachan BM, Harrow M, Adler D, et al: A checklist for the diagnosis of schizophrenia. Br J Psychiatry 12:529–539, 1972

Balant-Gorgia AE, Balant L: Antipsychotic drugs: clinical pharmacokinetics of potential candidates for plasma concentration monitoring. Clin Pharmacokinet 13:65–90, 1987

Baldessarini RJ, Cohen BM, Teicher NH: Significance of neuroleptic dose and plasma level in the pharmacological treatment of psychosis. Arch Gen Psychiatry 45:79–91, 1988

Casper R, Garver DL, Dekirmenjian H: Phenothiazine levels in plasma and red blood cells. Arch Gen Psychiatry 37:301–305, 1984

Chang SS, Javaid JI, Dysken MW, at al: Plasma levels of fluphenazine during fluphenazine decanoate treatment in schizophrenia. Psychopharmacology (Berl) 87:55–58, 1985

Cimbura G: Review of methods of analysis for phenothiazine drugs. J Chromatogr Sci 10:287–293, 1972

Cochran E, Carl J, Hanin I, et al: Effect of vacutainer stoppers on plasma tricyclic levels: a reevaluation. Commun Psychopharmacol 2:495–503, 1978

Cohen BM, Lipinski JF, Harris PQ, et al: Clinical use of the radioreceptor assay for neuroleptics. Psychiatry Res 1:173–178, 1980

Curry SH: Determination of nanogram quantities of chlorpromazine or its metabolites in plasma using gas liquid chromatography with an electron capture detector. Anal Chem 40:1251–1255, 1968

Curry SH: Antipsychotic drugs, I: chlorpromazine: pharmacokinetics, plasma levels, and clinical response, in Plasma Levels of Psychotropic Drugs and Clinical Response. Edited by Burrows GD, Norman TR. New York, Marcel Dekker, 1981, pp 243–286

Curry SH, Derr JE, Naling HM: The physiological disposition of chlorpromazine in the rat and dog. Proc Soc Exp Biol Med 134:314–318, 1970a

Curry SH, Marshall JH, Davis JM, et al: Chlorpromazine plasma levels and effects. Arch Gen Psychiatry 22:289–296, 1970b

Dahl SG: Plasma level monitoring of antipsychotic drugs. Clin Pharmacokinet 11:36–61, 1986

Davis JM, Ericksen SE, Hart S, et al: Haloperidol plasma levels and clinical response: basic concepts and clinical data. Psychopharmacol Bull 21:48–51, 1985

Dhar AK, Kutt H: Improved liquid-chromatographic determination of haloperidol in plasma. Clin Chem 30:1228–1230, 1984

Dysken MW, Javaid JI, Chang SS, et al: Fluphenazine pharmacokinetics and therapeutic response. Psychopharmacology (Berl) 73:205–210, 1981

Garver DL, Dekirmenjian H, Davis JM, et al: Neuroleptic drug levels and therapeutic response: preliminary observations with red blood cell bound butaperazine. Am J Psychiatry 134:304–307, 1977

Garver DL, Hirschowitz J, Glicksteen GA, et al: Haloperidol plasma and red blood cell levels and clinical antipsychotic response. J Clin Psychopharmacol 4:133–137, 1984

Hansen LB, Larsen NE, Gulmann N: Dose-response relationships of perphenazine in the treatment of acute psychoses. Psychopharmacology (Berl) 78:112–115, 1982

Hansen LB, Larsen, NE: Therapeutic advantage of monitoring plasma concentrations of perphenazine in clinical practice. Psychopharmacology (Berl) 87:16–19, 1985

Heyes WL, Salmon JR: Some aspects of the high-performance liquid chromatography of fluphenazine and its esters. J Chromatogr 156:309–316, 1978

Honigfeld G, Klett C: The Nurses' Observation Scale for Inpatient Evaluation (NOSIE): a new scale for measuring improvement in chronic schizophrenia. J Clin Psychol 21:65–71, 1965

Janicak PG, Javaid JI, Sharma RP, et al: Trifluoperazine plasma levels and clinical response. J Clin Psychopharmacol 9:340–346, 1989

Javaid JI, Pandey GN, Duslak B, et al: Measurement of neuroleptic concentrations by GLC and radioreceptor assay. Commun Psychopharmacol 4:467–475, 1980

Javaid JI, Dekirmenjian H, Liskevych U, et al: Fluphenazine determination in human plasma by a sensitive gas chromatographic method using nitrogen detector. J Chromatogr Sci 19:439–443, 1981

Javaid JI, Dekirmenjian H, Davis JM: GLC analysis of trifluoperazine in human plasma. J Pharm Sci 71:63–66, 1982a

Javaid JI, Linden RD, Davis JJ: Measurement of antipsychotics in patients. Psychopharm Bull 18:227–228, 1982b

Javaid JI, Janicak PG, Hedeker D, et al: Steady state plasma level prediction for haloperidol from a single test dose. Psychopharmacol Bull 27:83–87, 1991a

Javaid JI, Janicak PG, Holland, D: Blood level monitoring of antipsychotics and antidepressants. Psychiatr Med 9:163–187, 1991b

Jemal M, Ivashkiv E, Both D, et al: Picogram level determination of fluphenazine in human plasma by automated gas chromatography/mass selective detection. Biomed Environ Mass Spectrom 14:699–704, 1987

Jorgenson A: Metabolism and pharmacokinetics of antipsychotic drugs, in Progress in Drug Metabolism, Vol 9. Edited by Bridges JW, Chasseaud LF. Philadelphia, PA, Taylor and Francis, 1986, pp 111–174

Korpi ER, Kleinman JE, Costakos DT, et al: Reduced haloperidol in the post-mortem brains of haloperidol-treated patients. Psychiatry Res 11:259–269, 1984

Magliozzi JR, Hollister LE, Arnold KV, et al: Relationship of haloperidol levels to clinical response in schizophrenic patients. Am J Psychiatry 138:365–367, 1981

Marder SR, Van Putten T, Aravaziri M, et al: Fluphenazine plasma levels and clinical response. Psychopharmacol Bull 26:256–259, 1990

Mavroidis M, Kanter DR, Hirschowitz J, et al: Clinical response and plasma haloperidol levels in schizophrenia. Psychopharmacology 81:354–356, 1983

Mavroidis ML, Kantor DR, Hirschowitz J, et al: Clinical relevance of thiothixene plasma levels. J Clin Psychopharmacol 4:155–157, 1984

May PRA, Van Putten T, Jenden DJ, et al: Chlorpromazine levels and the outcome of treatment in schizophrenic patients. Arch Gen Psychiatry 38:202–207. 1981

National Institute of Mental Health: CGI (Clinical Global Impression) Scale. Psychopharmacol Bull 21:839–843, 1985

Overall JE, Gorham DR: The Brief Psychiatric Rating Scale. Psychol Rep 10:799–812, 1962

Perry PS, Pfohl BM, Kelly MW: The relationship of haloperidol concentrations to therapeutic response. J Clin Psychopharmacol 8:38–43, 1988

Potkin SG, Shen Y, Pardes H, et al: Does a therapeutic window for plasma haloperidol exist? Preliminary Chinese data. Psychopharmacol Bull 21:48–51, 1985

Santos JL, Cabranes JA, Vazquez C, et al: Clinical response and plasma haloperidol levels in chronic and subchronic schizophrenia. Biol Psychiatry 26:381–388, 1989

Schaffer CB, Shahid A, Javaid JI, et al: Bioavailability of intramuscular versus oral haloperidol in schizophrenic patients. J Clin Psychopharmacol 2:274–277, 1982

Shostak M, Perel JM, Stiller RL, et al: Plasma haloperidol and clinical response: a role for reduced haloperidol in antipsychotic activity? J Clin Psychopharmacol 7:394–400, 1987

Smith RC: Plasma haloperidol levels and clinical response. Arch Gen Psychiatry 44:1110–1112, 1987

Smith RC, Baumgartner R, Chandra MS, et al: Haloperidol. Arch Gen Psychiatry 41:1044–1049, 1984

Smith RC, Baumgartner R, Skvartsbard A, et al: Comparison efficacy of red cell and plasma haloperidol as predictors of clinical response in schizophrenia. Psychopharmacology (Berl) 85:449–455, 1985

Smith RC, Crayton J, Dekirmenjian H, et al: Blood levels of neuroleptic drugs in nonresponding chronic schizophrenic patients. Arch Gen Psychiatry 36:579-584, 1979

Spitzer RL, Gibson M, Endicott J: Global Assessment Scale. New York, New York State Department of Mental Hygiene, 1973

Spitzer RL, Endicott J, Robins E: Research Diagnostic Criteria: rationale and reliability. Arch Gen Psychiatry 325:773–782, 1978

Szczepanik-VanLeeuwen PA: Improved gas chromatographic-mass spectrometric assay for haloperidol utilizing ammonia chemical ionization and selected-ion monitoring. J Chromatogr 339:321–330, 1985

Van Putten T, Marder SR, May PRA, et al: Plasma level of haloperidol and clinical response. Psychopharmacol Bull 21:69–72, 1985

Van Putten T, Marder SR, Monty J, et al: Haloperidol plasma levels and clinical response: a therapeutic window relationship. Psychopharmacol Bull 24:172–175, 1988

Van Putten T, Aravagiri M, Marder S, et al: Plasma fluphenazine levels and clinical response in newly admitted schizophrenic patients. Psychopharmacol Bull 27:91–96, 1991

Volavka J, Cooper TB: Review of haloperidol level and clinical response: looking through the window. J Clin Psychopharmacol 7:25–30, 1987

Volavka J, Cooper TB, Czobor P, et al: Haloperidol blood levels and clinical effects. Arch Gen Psychiatry 49:354–361, 1992

White VR, Frings SS, Villairanca JE, et al: Rapid fluorometric determination of phenothiazines employing in situ photochemical oxidation. Anal Chem 48:1314–1316, 1976

Wiles DH, Franklin M: Radioimmunoassay for fluphenazine in human plasma. Br J Clin Pharmacol 5:265–268, 1979

Wode-Helgodt B, Borg S, Fyro B, et al: Clinical effects and drug concentrations in plasma and cerebrospinal fluid in psychotic patients treated with fixed doses of chlorpromazine. Acta Psychiatr Scand 58:149–173, 1978

Wurzburger RJ, Miller RL, Marcum EA, et al: A new radioimmunoassay for haloperidol. Direct measurement of serum and striatal concentrations. J Pharmacol Exp Ther 217:757–763, 1981

Yesavage JA, Holman CA, Cohn R, et al: Correlation of initial serum levels and clinical response. Arch Gen Psychiatry 40:301–304, 1983

CHAPTER 3

Fluphenazine Plasma Levels, Dose, and Acute Treatment Response

Douglas F. Levinson, M.D.
George M. Simpson, M.D.
E.-S. Lo, Ph.D.
Thomas B. Cooper, M.A.

Fluphenazine hydrochloride, a high-potency piperazine phenothiazine, was originally introduced over 30 years ago on the basis of uncontrolled, flexible-dose studies of diagnostically heterogeneous samples of patients. The manufacturer's package insert recommendation was for 2.5 to 10 mg/day in most cases, with a maximum up to 20 mg/day. Between 1961 and 1971, six blind, controlled studies established the efficacy of oral fluphenazine in the treatment of psychotic exacerbations. In fixed-dose studies, Howell et al. (1961) found fluphenazine 5 mg/day to be as effective as trifluoperazine 12.5 mg/day in 48 subjects treated for 2 weeks, and Clark et al. (1971) found fluphenazine 10 mg/day superior to placebo and as effective as chlorpromazine or thioridazine (1,000 mg/day each) in a 4-week study of 75 subjects. Four flexible-dose studies (Lasky et al. 1962; NIMH Collaborative Study Group 1964, 1967; Hanlon et al. 1965) (average daily doses of 5.9–10 mg) found fluphenazine to be as effective as comparable neuroleptics (e.g., chlorpromazine at average daily doses of 396–746 mg) and more effective than placebo (NIMH Collaborative Study Group 1964), thioridazine 193 mg/day (Hanlon et al. 1965), or reserpine 6 mg/day (Lasky et al. 1962). Although a next step might have been con-

This work was supported by NIMH Grant RO1 MH-41585 (to Dr. Simpson).

trolled dose-response and plasma level studies on diagnostically better-defined samples to optimize the ratio of therapeutic to adverse effects, such studies have been rare for neuroleptics generally.

Perhaps one reason for the dearth of controlled studies of doses in the usual clinical range was the realization that many chronically psychotic patients responded poorly to neuroleptic treatment. This led to the use of increasingly higher doses in the United States, and to several studies of very high doses of several drugs including fluphenazine. Quitkin et al. (1975) studied 6 weeks of oral fluphenazine (up to 1,200 mg/day vs. 30 mg/day) in poorly responsive patients, finding no advantage for the "megadose." In acute patients, Escobar et al. (1983) and Coffman et al. (1987) both reported no advantage to "rapid neuroleptization" with fluphenazine in controlled studies. Rifkin (1986) and Baldessarini et al. (1988) reviewed this literature and concluded that high-dose treatment offered no therapeutic advantage for acute or maintenance treatment. The dose pendulum then swung the other way as outpatient studies were beginning to demonstrate the efficacy of relatively low doses, e.g., of fluphenazine decanoate injections (Kane 1983; Marder et al. 1984). Baldessarini et al. (1988) concluded in an exhaustive review that the low-to-moderate dose range was most effective, but the review demonstrated that few controlled acute studies have compared multiple doses of the same drug within this range. Plasma level studies of other neuroleptics are reviewed elsewhere in this volume.

Early studies failed to establish a definitive relationship between plasma level and response but methodological problems were common, particularly a failure to randomly assign subjects to fixed dose regimens irrespective of clinical state (to prevent the clinician's impression of severity from influencing plasma level). Chlorpromazine, for example, did not show consistent plasma level–response relationships (Wode-Helgodt et al. 1978; reviewed by Dahl 1986), and proved to have an excessive number of active metabolites (Dahl 1986). The neuroleptic radioreceptor assay (RRA) method was developed in an attempt to measure all dopamine-2 receptor-blocking activity, but it was neither adequately sensitive nor predictive of response in most studies (reviewed by Midha et al. 1987). Fluphenazine presented an additional problem: plasma concentrations during treatment at effective doses are low (often < 1 ng/ml), and sufficiently sensitive and accurate assays did not become available until the 1980s. Many early methods such as gas-liquid chromatography (GLC) could not detect levels below 1–2 ng/ml (reviewed by Midha et al. 1980). A number of more sensitive methods have been developed: analytic methods (with lower limits of sensitivity shown in parentheses) have included gas chromatography (GC) with nitrogen detection (0.2 ng/ml; Javaid et al. 1981), high-performance liquid chromatography (HPLC) (0.2 ng/ml; Ereshefsky et al. 1983) and HPLC combined with radioimmunoassay (RIA) (0.16 ng/ml; Goldstein and Van Vunakis 1981), and high-performance thin-layer chromatography (0.1 ng/ml; Davis and Fenimore 1983). Two RIA methods are currently used in most clinical studies, both with good specificity and low coefficients of variation at low levels, with lower limits of sensitivity currently reported at 0.100 ng/ml (Midha 1980; see also Chapter 7 this volume) and 0.020 ng/ml (Lo et al. 1988).

Acute Treatment Studies of Fluphenazine Plasma Levels

There have been five reported studies of outcome in relation to fluphenazine plasma levels during acute treatment. The first three (Dysken et al. 1981; Mavroidis et al. 1984a, 1984b; Hitzemann et al. 1986) used a GC assay (Javaid et al. 1981) that detects 0.2 ng/ml but is linear only above 0.5 ng/ml; many subjects were reported having levels less than 0.5 ng/ml. Each of these three studies treated acute inpatients with fixed dosages of 5, 10, or 20 mg/day of oral fluphenazine for 2 weeks and examined the relationship of plasma levels to percent improvement in versions of the New Haven Schizophrenia Index (NHSI; Astrachan et al. 1972) rating scale. Raters were blind to plasma levels but otherwise dose was apparently open. The fourth study (Van Putten et al. 1991) used a more sensitive RIA method, as did our study, which will be discussed further below. (Studies of chronic fluphenazine treatment are reviewed in Chapter 7.)

Dysken et al. (1981) studied 29 schizophrenic or schizoaffective patients by Research Diagnostic Criteria (RDC; Spitzer et al. 1981). Doses were predetermined but not random (5 or 10 mg/day in some initial subjects, 20 mg/day in most). The authors suggested a "therapeutic window" effect because three patients with plasma levels greater than 2.8 ng/ml and three with levels less than 0.2 ng/ml all showed poor response. The conclusion is limited, however, by the small number of subjects with levels outside the therapeutic window, the dependence of the statistical effect on three "outliers" with very high plasma levels, and the number of subjects ($n = 12$) with levels below 0.5 ng/ml (the reliably linear range of the assay).

Mavroidis et al. (1984a, 1984b) randomly assigned 19 schizophrenic inpatients as defined by DSM-III (American Psychiatric Association 1980) to the above-mentioned doses. A significant curvilinear relationship was found between fluphenazine plasma level and percent improvement in the NHSI, with 45% symptom reduction (the predetermined criterion for response) associated with plasma levels of 0.13 to 0.70 ng/ml. No subjects had plasma levels below the "minimum" value of 0.13 ng/ml, and 5 of the 19 subjects had levels of less than 0.5 ng/ml. The 11 subjects with plasma levels greater than 0.70 ng/ml had significantly less improvement than those with lower levels.

The same group (Hitzemann et al. 1986) treated 15 schizophrenic inpatients (as defined by DSM-III) with "predetermined" fixed dosages (5, 10, or 20 mg/day). In addition to the GC fluphenazine assay, they used a modified RRA with somewhat high coefficients of variation (14%–26%). The two assays differed to a variable extent, with the RRA generally showing higher levels. The relationship between fluphenazine plasma level and outcome was not described; presumably it was not significant. For RRA, no therapeutic window was found, but based on a complex analysis, it was concluded that there were two subgroups, one responding to low levels (RRA equivalent to 0.19 to 0.91 ng/ml fluphenazine), and the other to higher levels (> 2.5 ng/ml). There were four responsive patients in each of these two groups.

Van Putten et al. (1991) treated 72 exacerbated male schizophrenic inpatients (as defined by DSM-III) for 4 weeks, apparently openly, with 5, 10, or 20 mg/day of oral fluphenazine. Fluphenazine levels were assayed by RIA with a sensitivity of 0.100 ng/ml (Midha et al. 1980). The results were analyzed by logistic regression in terms of two outcome measures: the proportion of subjects in a given plasma level range showing moderate or marked global clinical improvement and/or "disabling [subjectively unbearable] side effects." In patients with plasma levels in the range of 0.5–1.5 ng/ml, approximately 55%–65% improved but 30%–45% had disabling side effects. A lower proportion of responsive patients (20%) with modest side effects had blood plasma levels below this range and a high proportion of both responsiveness and disabling side effects (both about 90%) with blood plasma levels above it. The largest proportion of subjects who improved without disabling side effects had blood plasma levels in the vicinity of 0.4–0.8 ng/ml, although improvement was more likely above this range. The same group (Van Putten et al. 1991) studied chronic treatment with fluphenazine decanoate using the same assay. They found a high risk of exacerbation at levels below 0.5 ng/ml, less risk through the range of 0.8–1.0 ng/ml, and very low risk above 2 ng/ml. Thus the therapeutic effects of fluphenazine seemed to occur in approximately the same plasma level range with two forms of the drug in both acute and chronic treatment.

A Study of Fluphenazine Plasma Levels and Dose During Acute Treatment

Our study (Sramek et al. 1988) was designed to address the methodological issues that have been raised about psychotropic plasma level studies including diagnosis by a structured instrument and specified criteria, randomized and fixed dose schedules, double-blind dose assignment, an adequate treatment period, and sensitive drug assay. Preliminary analyses including the majority of subjects are discussed here.

Subjects

The subjects were inpatients newly admitted for exacerbations of psychosis. The setting was the acute unit of a university hospital receiving referrals from community mental health centers. All subjects had not been taking major psychotropic drugs for at least 5–7 days and usually for a month or more. They were interviewed by using the Schedule for Affective Disorders and Schizophrenia (SADS; Endicott and Spitzer 1978, and diagnosed by RDC and DSM-III-R (American Psychiatric Association 1987) criteria based on all available sources of information. Patients were invited to participate if they met criteria for RDC definite or probable schizophrenia or schizoaffective disorder (mainly schizophrenic subtype), and did not have an organic mental disorder, need for concurrent nonpsychiatric medications with central nervous systems effects, primary mental retardation, toxic psychosis, or a history of resistance to neuroleptic treatment (two previous trials at specified doses without improvement).

These subjects were fairly typical of the diverse types of patients seen in community settings. In order to account for the effects of diagnostic "purity" without limiting the sample size excessively, we subdivided subjects into two groups: those with definite RDC schizophrenia or schizoaffective (mainly schizophrenic subtype) diagnoses of a minimum 6-month duration with no atypical or complicating features, and those with complicating features (see details in Levinson et al. 1990). Of the 53 patients who completed the study, 34 had uncomplicated diagnoses (24 schizophrenic, 5 schizoaffective manic, and 5 schizoaffective depressed), and 19 had complicating features (4 with RDC atypical clinical features such as borderline/histrionic features or childhood onset, 5 with IQs of 60–70, 11 with significant past substance abuse without current toxic psychosis, and 1 with previous head trauma without known sequelae but near the time of onset). Dose-response results were similar for these two groups so they were combined for this discussion. There were also 27 subjects who dropped out during this period, mostly because of withdrawal from treatment of unco-operative subjects with histories of substance abuse or atypical features, and less frequently because of extrapyramidal side effects or clinical worsening. They did not differ from the individuals who completed the study in drug dose or plasma level.

Methods and Procedure

After giving signed, informed consent, patients were interviewed for diag-nosis and rated by using the Brief Psychiatric Rating Scale (BPRS; Overall and Gorham 1962), a modified Simpson Neurological Rating Scale (NRS; Simpson and Angus 1970) for extrapyramidal symptoms (EPS), the Simp-son Tardive Dyskinesia Rating Scale (TDRS; Simpson et al. 1979), and the Schedule for Assessment of Negative Symptoms (SANS; Andreasen 1982). They were then assigned to a dose schedule (based on a random number table) by a pharmacist. Two different dose schedules were used during the course of the study. The first 23 patients who completed the study were treated for 24 days with 10 or 20 mg/day of oral fluphenazine, whereas the other 30 patients who completed the study received 28 days of treatment at 10, 20, or 30 mg/day. All subjects received an initial 5-mg dose on day 1, 1 or 2 days of dose escalation, and the full dosage thereafter (divided into two equal daily doses). Look-alike placebo tablets were administered by the pharmacist so that all subjects received the same number of tablets per dose. The only concurrent psychotropic drugs permitted were benztropine (for emergent EPS), chloral hydrate for sleep or mild agitation, and a lim-ited number of doses of amobarbital sodium for severe agitation.

Because all significant improvement occurred during the first three weeks of treatment, and because the groups treated by the two dose sched-ules showed the same relationships between outcome and dose or plasma level, the two groups were combined for analysis of end-of-study outcome. Blood for fluphenazine plasma level determinations was drawn at 9 A.M. (12 hours after the last dose). Fluphenazine was assayed by extraction RIA with a sensitivity of 20 pg/ml, with low split-sample coefficients of variation (e.g., 5% at 0.316–0.420 ng/ml and 8% at 0.081–0.110 ng/ml) (Lo et al. 1988). Measurements included in the present analyses were

+ Log of dose per unit weight (mg/kg per day), referred to as "dose"
+ Log of steady-state fluphenazine plasma level (ng/ml; mean of last two levels drawn), referred to as "plasma level"

✦ Percent improvement in BPRS-positive symptoms (sum of hallucinatory behavior, unusual thought content, and conceptual disorganization) from baseline to end of study (day 24 or 28), with each item rated on a scale of 0–6 so that complete remission of symptoms resulting in a score of 100% improvement (note that many studies use a 1–7 scale)
✦ Percent improvement of negative symptoms (sum of the five global items of the SANS from baseline to end of study, again on a scale of 0–6
✦ Maximum NRS score before any treatment with benztropine, excluding subjects who were treated for early dystonic reactions (Singh et al. 1990). The akathisia item was subtracted from the NRS and analyzed separately.

Results

A preliminary analysis (Levinson et al. 1988) of some of these subjects suggested that the strongest relationship between plasma level and improvement was seen in those subjects in whom positive symptoms decreased more than an arbitrary amount (50%). Therefore, the effects of dose were analyzed similarly (Levinson et al. 1990). For all subjects, dose did not predict response (percent improvement), but among the more responsive patients, a strong relationship was seen between improvement (for positive symptoms only) and dose. This was true whether the threshold was 50% or 40% but not lower. The 40% threshold was therefore adopted as a cutoff threshold to form a larger subgroup for analysis. Here we describe analyses of both plasma level and dose. There were 53 subjects available for analysis of dose, but only 49 subjects had valid steady-state plasma levels.

Plasma level and dose were correlated at $r = .51$ ($N = 49$, $P < .001$). Results for clinical improvement are shown in Figure 3–1. Two main multiple regression analyses were carried out. First, for the sample as a whole ($N = 49$), an overall multivariate statistical analysis showed no significant prediction of improvement by dose and plasma level (Wilks' lamda = 0.931, F [2,46] = 1.696, NS). The univariate F tests showed a possible weak relationship between plasma level and improvement ($P = .074$), but the multivariate statistic must be considered the more conservative test here.

Second, for subjects with improvement greater than 40% ($n = 26$), multivariate analysis did show a significant prediction of improvement by plasma level and dose (Wilks' lamda = 0.589, $F = 8.04$, $P = .002$). Univariate results showed a significant effect both for plasma level ($r = .44$, $P = .025$) and dose ($r = .64$, $P < .001$). In a stepwise regression procedure, plasma level added nothing to the predictive power of dose (partial correlation = – .05,

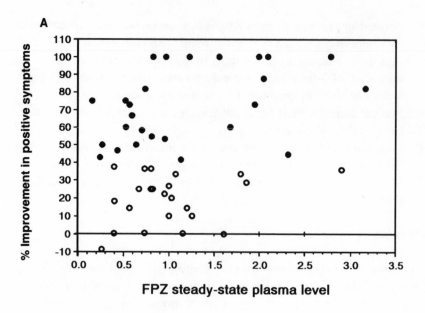

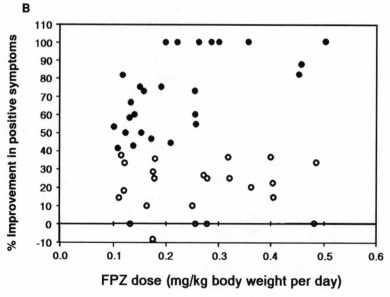

Figure 3–1. Relationship between fluphenazine steady- state plasma levels (ng/ml; *panel A*) or dosage (mg/kg body weight per day; *panel B*) and percent improvement in Brief Psychiatric Rating Scale (BPRS; Overall and Gorham 1962) positive symptoms from baseline to end of study. Solid circles represent subjects with greater than 40% reduction in positive symptoms during the study; open circles represent subjects with less than 40% improvement.

NS). However, analyses of covariance demonstrated that each variable predicted improvement in this subgroup even when the effects of the other variables were removed by covariance.

These results raised the question of whether plasma level might predict outcome in those patients who had received an "adequate" dose. In previous analyses (Levinson et al. 1990), responsive patients showed the greatest improvement with doses greater than 0.2 mg/kg. In our study, subjects with doses in that range (regardless of response) were examined (in a multiple regression with both dose and plasma level as predictors). The overall multivariate test ($n = 26$, Wilks' lamda = 0.775, $F[2,23] = 3.34$, $P = .053$) confirmed a trend toward higher plasma levels in subjects with greater improvement.

Other analyses (Levinson et al. 1992) of these data have shown significant improvement during the first 4–5 days, with responsive and nonresponsive patients differing in improvement only at 2 weeks and beyond. Significant improvement occurred through 3 weeks, with slower (not statistically significant) further improvement during the fourth week.

EPS correlated with dose at $r = .51$ ($n = 31$, $P = .003$), but only weakly with plasma level ($n = 31$, $r = .34$, $P = .06$; Figure 3–2). EPS scores did not correlate with improvement. The presence of akathisia at any point predicted that improvement would be less than 40% ($n = 47$, $F[1,45] = 20.097$, $P < .001$); the only similar predictor was longer duration of illness (Levinson et al. 1990). The few patients with akathisia who obtained significant relief from anticholinergic agents (too few for analysis) still seemed to have a poor clinical outcome. Presence of akathisia was weakly predicted by dose ($P = .068$) but not by plasma level.

Discussion

The results of our study to date, and those of Van Putten et al. (1991) permit some tentative conclusions about fluphenazine plasma levels during acute treatment. The most cautious interpretation of our study would be that neither dose nor plasma level can predict improvement during 4 weeks of treatment. A second possibility is that the dose range we studied was too narrow (our lowest dose of 10 mg/day was higher than doses shown to be superior to placebo in some of the early studies cited above) to allow us to define a lower threshold for acute effects. (It is of historical interest that in 1983, when this study was designed, high-dose neuroleptic treatment was common, and we seriously wondered whether hospital staff would balk at

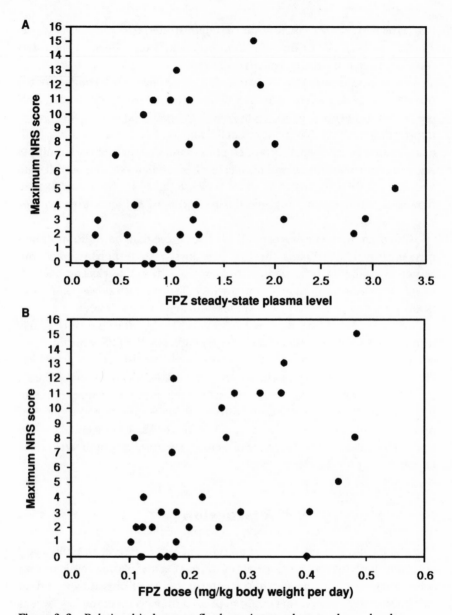

Figure 3–2. Relationship between fluphenazine steady-state plasma levels (ng/ml; *panel A*) or dosage (mg/kg body weight per day; *panel B*) and maximum Neurological Rating Scale (NRS; Simpson and Angus 1970) score (measuring extrapyramidal symptoms [EPS] with the akathisia item subtracted from the score) before initiation of antiparkinson agents. Subjects who were treated for dystonic reactions have been excluded because they received benztropine before maximum EPS would be expected to appear.

a dose as low as 10 mg/day.) The results of the study suggest that doses around 10 mg/day (between 0.1 and 0.2 mg/kg body weight per day) and plasma levels over 0.4 ng/ml are sufficient to produce at least a recognizable antipsychotic response in many neuroleptic-responsive patients (defined here as 40% reduction in ratings of psychotic symptoms), with relatively modest EPS. The assumption that the minimal threshold for response is below 0.4 ng/ml is supported by the study of Van Putten et al. (1991) where the lowest dose was 5 mg/day, and the one-eighth of subjects whose plasma levels clustered around 0.25 ng/ml showed a poor response.

We suggest that the subgroup that exceeded the criterion of response can provide additional information. Clinicians are most interested in providing "optimal" rather than "minimal" treatment. The analysis of rates of response (i.e., proportions of patients improving more than a minimum threshold), although typical in neuroleptic studies, fails to give information about the maximal amount of response. For this reason, we have emphasized the prediction of the percent reduction in ratings of neuroleptic target symptoms (hallucinations, delusions, and thought disorder), and found this to be related to dose and plasma level only in subjects with at least 40% reduction in positive symptoms.

It is generally agreed that treatment-resistant patients should be excluded from this type of study because neuroleptic response is so variable in schizophrenia that it is difficult to determine whether treatment factors (such as dose or plasma level) or illness factors are responsible for a patient's improvement or lack of it. In practice, exclusion of all non-responsive patients is difficult. One can study recent-onset, very acute (and usually responsive) patients, but there may be spontaneous remissions in this group, and the findings might also be difficult to generalize to the majority of patients. One can exclude patients with known histories of neuroleptic resistance, as in our study, but as shown here, this does not eliminate many of the patients who ultimately fail to respond to the study drug in the available time period.

Outpatient neuroleptic studies have an advantage in addressing this issue. In one common design, recently remitted patients are "stabilized" on neuroleptics for some months, and then randomly assigned to maintenance treatments. This design selects subjects known to be vulnerable to relapse and to be much less symptomatic on neuroleptics. They are thus at high risk of relapse on inadequate doses, maximizing the power of the study. A comparable sample for an acute study would be patients who had previously been observed to respond to the study drug but who then chose to discontinue the drug, subsequently relapsed, and (before other treatments could be instituted) agreed to participate in a double-blind study of a wide range of randomized doses. It would probably also be preferable to exclude subjects with very short or very long durations of illness. The problems inherent in finding such a sample are obvious.

Our approach attempts to achieve at least part of the goal of focusing on treatment-responsive patients. Analysis of patients who meet a minimum criterion of improvement during the period of study should exclude at least some subjects in whom dose and plasma level is unrelated to short-term improvement, that is, those who fail to response either to the study drug or to any drug, and those who need longer periods of treatment to show minimal response. It fails to exclude the few who remit spontaneously. It presumably does exclude some subjects who failed to respond because of ineffective dose or plasma level; thus this approach will not identify the minimal threshold of response. It should succeed, however, in increasing the study's power to identify, within the most improved subgroup, any strong relationship between plasma level or dose and a quantitative measure of response and to identify treatment factors associated with maximal improvement. Other investigators have not reported attempts to replicate this strategy, which requires

◆ Data from a fixed-dose regimen, fixed-treatment period, preferably double-blind study
◆ Exclusion of subjects who failed to meet a minimal criterion of improvement during the study period (regardless of the eventual response)
◆ Use of a measure of improvement in specific target symptoms quantitating the range from complete to modest remission.

In our study, both dose and plasma level were predictive of outcome in the more improved subgroup. Dose was a better predictor than plasma level, but the difference between the two correlations with outcome was not significant. (Furthermore, plasma level showed a weak relationship with outcome for the entire sample.) We suggest that there is a sigmoidal dose-response function for acute fluphenazine treatment, that available dose, plasma level and improvement measures are imprecise indexes of this function, and that dose and plasma level can be helpful in guiding treatment. Measurements of metabolites might refine predictions based on plasma levels, but this has not generally been the case for psychotropics. Marder and colleagues (Aravagiri et al. 1990) are currently studying this issue for fluphenazine.

Possible guidelines can be derived from the linear regression coefficients identified in our improved subgroup. A 40% reduction in positive symptoms would be predicted in responsive patients at a plasma level of 0.55 ng/ml, and a dose of 0.13 mg/kg body weight per day, whereas an 80% reduction would be predicted at 1.05 ng/ml and 0.225 mg/kg body weight per day. These plasma level estimates are in the same range as those of Van Putten et al. (1991) for both acute and chronic treatment; their chronic treatment data are particularly useful here, because a 4-week study cannot determine response to lower plasma levels or doses for longer periods of time. Van Putten et al. (1991) demonstrated a high relapse rate among patients treated chronically at plasma levels much below 0.8–1.0 ng/ml.

For acute treatment with oral fluphenazine, dose may be as valuable as plasma levels in most cases. Treatment with 0.1–0.2 mg/kg body weight per day (5–15 mg/day for most patients) would be expected to produce at least minimal remission in most fluphenazine-responsive patients, with mild EPS except in particularly vulnerable patients. Treatment in the range of 0.2–0.25 mg/kg body weight per day (10–20 mg/day for most patients) is probably optimal for most responsive patients, with marked reduction in positive symptoms and mild to moderate EPS. For patients with a documented history of poor response (including those with akathisia), this latter range probably offers more side effects and little therapeutic advantage over lower doses. Although antipsychotic effects for responsive patients are quite substantial at 0.3 mg/kg body weight per day or more, EPS are likely to be quite severe in many cases. We would suggest, however, that fluphenazine plasma level measurements, if routinely available, would offer a number of benefits for many patients including:

✦ Maximal symptom reduction during acute treatment appears most likely to occur at plasma levels of approximately 1–2 ng/ml, with side effects typically increasing from moderate to more severe within this range. This range is likely to be associated with doses of 0.2–0.3 mg/kg body weight per day, but plasma levels could be useful in individualizing doses according to clinical priorities (symptom reduction versus severity of EPS).

✦ For patients with severe side effects, or those reluctant to take medication, titration of plasma levels to 0.5–0.8 ng/ml (typically at doses of about 0.15 mg/kg body weight per day) would probably result in some degree of remission with minimal or mild EPS.

✦ An acute plasma level would serve as a baseline to guide future treatment with fluphenazine decanoate (given the similarity in plasma level findings for the two drugs), following the recommendations of Van Putten et al. (1991): levels around 0.8–0.9 ng/ml for typical maintenance, and over 1.2 ng/ml for maximum protection from relapse.

✦ Plasma levels permit detection of noncompliance (very low or widely fluctuating levels) and of unusually high or low plasma levels.

A similar approach might be possible with haloperidol (Van Putten et al. 1991), although the data remain controversial (Volavka et al. 1990), and possibly perphenazine (reviewed in Van Putten et al. 1991). Such an approach would provide a more rational basis for treatment. Currently, neuroleptics are often prescribed based on biases for low versus high doses. Plasma levels could provide feedback to help the clinician assess the effects of dose changes in patients without risking the use of either excessively high or excessively low levels. This might encourage greater efforts, over time, to work with patients to identify optimal doses. We believe that this would result in both more conservative and more effective treatment for many patients. Clinicians should note, however, that to the best of our knowledge, sensitive RIA determinations of fluphenazine are not yet commercially available .

Finally, the relationship between akathisia and poor response deserves further study (Levinson et al. 1990). Akathisia was not well predicted by either dose or plasma level and thus might be a manifestation of an independent underlying mechanism involved in response to neuroleptics. Although the poor outcome associated with akathisia might simply be a result of the associated discomfort, it is our impression that this is not the case based on the variability of the reported subjective discomfort and the poor clinical outcome observed in some patients whose akathisia resolved on anticholinergic treatment.

References

American Psychiatric Association: Diagnostic and Statistical Manual of Mental Disorders, 3rd Edition. Washington, DC, American Psychiatric Association, 1980

American Psychiatric Association: Diagnostic and Statistical Manual of Mental Disorders, 3rd Edition, Revised. Washington, DC, American Psychiatric Association, 1987

Andreasen NC: Negative symptoms in schizophrenia: definition and reliability. Arch Gen Psychiatry 39:784–788, 1982

Aravagiri M, Marder SR, Van Putten T, et al: Therapeutic monitoring of steady-state plasma levels of the N-4-oxide metabolite of fluphenazine in chronically treated schizophrenic patients determined by a specific and sensitive radioimmunoassay. Ther Drug Monit 12:268–276, 1990

Astrachan BM, Harrow M, Adler D, et al: A checklist for the diagnosis of schizophrenia. Br J Psychiatry 121:529–539, 1972

Baldessarini RJ, Cohen BM, Teicher MH: Significance of neuroleptic dose and plasma level in the pharmacological treatment of psychoses. Arch Gen Psychiatry 45:79–91, 1988

Clark ML, Huber WK, Charalampous KD, et al: Drug treatment in newly admitted schizophrenic patients. Arch Gen Psychiatry 25:404–409, 1971

Coffman JA, Nasrallah HA, Lyskowski J, et al: Clinical effectiveness of oral and parenteral rapid neuroleptization. J Clin Psychiatry 48:20–24, 1987

Dahl SG: Plasma level monitoring of antipsychotic drugs. Clinical utility. Clin Pharmacokinet 11:36–61, 1986

Davis CM, Fenimore DC: Determination of fluphenazine in plasma by high-performance thin-layer chromatography. J Chromatogr 272:157–165, 1983

Dysken MW, Javaid JI, Chang SS, et al.: Fluphenazine pharmacokinetics and therapeutic response. Psychopharmacology (Berl) 73:205–210, 1981

Endicott J, Spitzer RL: A diagnostic interview: the schedule for affective disorders and schizophrenia. Arch Gen Psychiatry 35:837–844, 1978

Ereshefsky L, Saklad SR, Jann MW, et al: Pharmacokinetics of fluphenazine (FPZ) by high performance thin layer chromatography. Drug Intell Clin Pharm 17:436–437, 1983

Escobar JI, Barron A, Kiriakos R: A controlled study of neuroleptization with fluphenazine hydrochloride injections. J Clin Psychopharmacol 3:359–362, 1983

Goldstein SA, Van Vunakis H: Determination of fluphenazine, related phenothiazine drugs and metabolites by combined high-performance liquid chromatography and radioimmunoassay. J Pharmacol Exp Ther 217:36–43, 1981

Hanlon TE, Michaux MH, Ota KY, et al: The comparative effectiveness of eight phenothiazines. Psychopharmacologia 7:89–106, 1965

Hitzemann RJ, Garver DL, Mavroidis M, et al: Fluphenazine activity and antipsychotic response. Psychopharmacology (Berl) 90:270–273, 1986

Howell RJ, Brown HM, Beahgler ME: A comparison of fluphenazine, trifluoperazine and a placebo in the context of an active treatment unit. J Nerv Ment Dis 132:522–530, 1961

Javaid JI, Dekirmenjian H, Liskevych U, et al: Fluphenazine determination in human plasma by a sensitive gas chromatographic method using nitrogen detector. J Chromatogr Sci 19:439–443, 1981

Kane JM: Low dose medication strategies in the maintenance treatment of schizophrenia. Schizophr Bull 9:528–532, 1983

Lasky JJ, Klett CJ, Caffey EM, et al: Drug treatment of schizophrenic patients. Dis Nerv Syst 23:698–706, 1962

Levinson DF, Simpson GM, Singh H, et al: Neuroleptic plasma level may predict response in patients who meet a criterion for improvement. Arch Gen Psychiatry 45:878–879, 1988

Levinson DF, Simpson GM, Singh H, et al: Fluphenazine dose, clinical response, and extrapyramidal symptoms during acute treatment. Arch Gen Psychiatry 47:761–768, 1990

Levinson DF, Singh H, Simpson GM: Timing of acute clinical response to fluphenazine: A controlled study. Br J Psychiatry 160:365–371, 1992

Lo ES, Fein M, Hunter C, et al: A highly sensitive and specific radioimmunoassay for quantitation of plasma fluphenazine. J Pharm Sci 77:255–258, 1988

Marder SR, Van Putten T, Mintz J, et al: Costs and benefits of two doses of fluphenazine. Arch Gen Psychiatry 41:1025–1029, 1984

Mavroidis ML, Kanter DR, Hirschowitz J, et al: Therapeutic blood levels of fluphenazine: plasma or RBC determinations? Psychopharmacol Bull 20:168–170, 1984a

Mavroidis ML, Kanter DR, Hirschowitz J, et al: Fluphenazine plasma levels and clinical response. J Clin Psychiatry 45:370–373, 1984b

Midha KK, Cooper JK, Hubbard JW: Radioimmunoassay for fluphenazine in human plasma. Commun Psychopharmacol 4:107–114, 1980

Midha KK, Hawes EM, Hubbard JW, et al: The search for correlations between neuroleptic plasma levels and clinical outcome: a critical review, in Psychopharmacology: The Third Generation of Progress. Edited by Meltzer HY. New York, Raven 1987, pp 1341–1351

National Institute of Mental Health Psychopharmacology Service Center Collaborative Study Group: Phenothiazine treatment in acute schizophrenia. Arch Gen Psychiatry 10:246–261, 1964

National Institute of Mental Health Psychopharmacology Research Branch Collaborative Study Group: differences in clinical effects of three phenothiazines in "acute" schizophrenia. Dis Nerv System 28:369–383, 1967

Overall JE, Gorham DP: The brief psychiatric rating scale (BPRS). Psychol Rep 10:799–812, 1962

Quitkin F, Rifkin A, Klein DF: A very high dosage vs standard dosage fluphenazine in schizophrenia. Arch Gen Psychiatry 32:1276–1281, 1975

Rifkin A: Neuroleptic dosage strategies in schizophrenia. International Drug Therapy Newsletter 21:17–20, 1986

Simpson GM, Angus JWS: A rating scale for extrapyramidal side-effects. Acta Psychiatr Scand Suppl 212:11–19, 1970

Simpson GM, Lee JH, Zoubok B, et al: A rating scale for tardive dyskinesia. Psychopharmacology (Berl) 64:171–179, 1979

Singh H, Levinson DF, Simpson GM, et al: Acute dystonia during fixed-dose neuroleptic treatment. J Clin Psychopharmol 10:389–396, 1990

Spitzer RL, Endicott J, Robins E: Research Diagnostic Criteria (RDC) for a selected group of functional disorders. New York, New York State Psychiatric Institute, Biometrics Research, 1981

Sramek JJ, Potkin SG, Hahn R: Neuroleptic plasma concentrations and clinical response: in search of a therapeutic window. Drug Intell Clin Pharm 22:373–380, 1988

Van Putten T, Marder SR, Wirshing WC, et al: Neuroleptic plasma levels. Schizophr Bull 17:197–216, 1991

Volavka J, Cooper TB, Meisner M, et al: Haloperidol blood levels and effects in schizophrenia and schizoaffective disorder: A progress report. Psychopharmacol Bull 26:13–17, 1990

Wode-Helgodt B, Borg S, Fyro B, et al: Clinical effects and drug concentrations in plasma and cerebrospinal fluid in psychotic patients treated with fixed doses of chlorpromazine. Acta Psychiatr Scand 58:149–173, 1978

Haloperidol Plasma Levels and Clinical Response

Theodore Van Putten, M.D.
Stephen R. Marder, M.D.

Most work on the relation between plasma levels of neuroleptics and clinical response has been done with haloperidol. Table 4–1 summarizes fixed-dose studies done with haloperidol. Four of those studies suggest a "therapeutic window" relationship between plasma haloperidol and clinical response. The suggested therapeutic ranges are: 6.5–16 ng/ml (Smith et al. 1984); 4–11 ng/ml (Mavroidis et al. 1983); 4–22 ng/ml (Potkin et al. 1985); and 12–55 ng/ml (Santos et al. 1989). The therapeutic range used by Santos et al. (1989) of 12–55 ng/ml is higher and inconsistent with the therapeutic ranges of the aforementioned three studies. Inspection of Santos et al.'s (1989) data indicates a positive linear relationship between approximately 2 ng/ml and 20 ng/ml, with a plateau relationship starting at 20 ng/ml. (Recalculation of Santos et al.'s data using two sigmoidal dose-effect functions [see section titled "Data Analysis"] indicates a plateau relationship starting at +19 ng/ml, and logarithmic conversion of plasma haloperidol levels suggests a plateau relationship starting at +18 ng/ml).

Six fixed-dose studies did not find a therapeutic-window relationship; however, this discrepancy may be explained by important features of these studies. Three studies used primarily patients who responded poorly to neuroleptics (Bigelow et al. 1985; Rimon et al. 1981; Itoh et al. 1984) and three studies used relatively low drug doses (5 mg/day or 10 mg/day, Bleeker et al. 1984; 6 mg/day, Itoh et al. 1984; 0.2 mg/kg body weight per day, Wistedt et al. 1984). As a result, the detection of an upper toxic limit was unlikely. Three studies used doses that were relatively high (60 mg/day and

Table 4–1. Fixed-dose studies of haloperidol

Study	N	Dose	Treatment duration (weeks)	Patient sample	Haloperidol window (ng/ml) or other relationship
Bleeker et al. (1984)	29	5 or 10 mg/day	2	Atypical and brief reactive psychosis	None
Potkin et al. (1985)	43	0.40 or 0.15 mg/kg body weight per day	6	Chinese schizophrenic patients	4.0–26.0
Bigelow et al. (1985)	19	0.40 mg/kg body weight per day	6	Institutionalized poor "responders"	None
Rimon et al. (1981)	12	60 and 120 mg/day	8	Institutionalized poor "responders"	None
Smith et al. (1984a)	27	10, 20, or 25 mg/day	3	Newly admitted schizophrenic patients	7.0–17.0, with poor "responders" excluded
Mavroidis et al. (1983)	14	6, 12, or 24 mg/day	2	Newly admitted DSM-III schizophrenic patients in psychotic exacerbation	4.7–11.0
Wistedt et al. (1984)	10	0.2 mg/kg body weight per day	4	"Acute schizophrenic patients"	Linear
Itoh et al. (1984)	11	6 mg/day	4	Institutionalized chronic schizophrenic patients	None
Linkowski et al. (1984)	20	30 mg/day	6	6 acute, 8 subacute, 6 subchronic newly admitted schizophrenic patients	None
Santos et al. (1989)	30	10, 15, or 30 mg/day	3	Nonresponsive, schizophreniform, schizoaffective patients excluded	12–55

120 mg/day, Rimon et al. 1981; 0.4 mg/kg body weight per day, Bigelow et al. 1985; 30 mg/day, Linkowski et al. 1984); therefore, patients were unlikely to have plasma levels in the subtherapeutic range. In retrospect, of the 10 fixed-dose studies with haloperidol, 4 were designed properly and all 4 found a therapeutic-window relationship.

In the studies (Smith et al. 1984; Mavroidis et al. 1983; Potkin et al. 1985; Santos et al. 1989) that suggested a therapeutic range, there are only 25 patients that define the proposed toxic range and 17 of these patients were in Potkin et al.'s (1985) investigation of Chinese schizophrenic patients in which the curvilinear fit explained only 8% of the variance of clinical improvement. Further, these studies lack the clinically obvious—what is the clinical state of patients with toxic haloperidol levels? Do patients with toxic plasma levels improve when their plasma levels are lowered and the converse? Only Mavroidis et al. (1983) mentioned that when they halved the dose in the patient with the highest plasma level (18.5 ng/ml) and little clinical improvement (11%), the patient improved "dramatically."

In two studies patients were randomly assigned to predetermined plasma haloperidol ranges. Volavka et al. (1990) assigned 152 schizophrenic inpatients to three fixed haloperidol plasma level ranges: low (2–13 ng/ml), medium (13.1–24 ng/ml), and high (24.1–35 ng/ml). Patients were rated on the Brief Psychiatric Rating Scale (BPRS; Overall and Gorham 1962) and the Simpson-Angus Scale (Simpson and Angus 1970) for side effects with investigators blind to the patient's plasma level. No significant differences were detected among any of the three haloperidol plasma level range assignment groups in side effects, drop-out rate, BPRS raw score, or categorical improvement.

Coryell et al. (1990) assigned 25 newly admitted psychotic patients (17 with schizophrenia; 4 with schizoaffective disorder, mainly schizophrenic; and 4 with unspecified functional psychosis) to two plasma level ranges: a "high" group (20–35 ng/ml) or a "medium" group (8–18 ng/ml). During 4 weeks of treatment, patients with plasma levels less than 18 ng/ml had a better outcome in terms of total BPRS score, as well as on positive and negative symptom scores. The relationship between plasma level and outcome was most powerful for the first week of treatment. Using a BPRS total score of 40 or less as an indicator of global improvement, 45% of patients in the "medium" plasma level range improved versus none of the patients in the higher plasma level range ($P = .005$).

In summary, there is evidence for a therapeutic window-type relationship with haloperidol in the acutely exacerbated patient but the evidence is not strong. Some chronic, neuroleptic-resistant patients seem to be able to tolerate high plasma levels, possibly without a deterioration of response. The utility of high plasma haloperidol levels (Van Putten et al. 1985) in neuroleptic-resistant patients is an unresearched area.

A New Study With Haloperidol

Sixty-nine newly readmitted drug-free (for at least 2 weeks, but usually several months) schizophrenic (by DSM-III criteria; American Psychiatric Association 1980) men were randomly assigned to receive haloperidol in doses of either 5, 10, or 20 mg daily for 4 weeks (Van Putten et al. 1990). In cases of no response, the physician could increase (or decrease) the dose for another 4 weeks depending on his or her clinical judgment. Clinical response was measured at baseline and weekly for the first 4 weeks, and at week 8 after the flexible-dose period. Clinical ratings were determined by investigators blind about patients' plasma levels.

On average, these patients were in their early thirties and had four previous hospitalizations. They had all served in the armed forces, had worked for 4.5 years at some time in their life, were judged "markedly ill" on a nurses' rating scale, and all scored at least "moderate" on conceptual disorganization, unusual thought content, or hallucinatory behavior. In fact, their mean baseline BPRS schizophrenia factor score was 13 (normal = 3, maximum = 21), indicating that they were quite psychotic at baseline. The very excited or menacing were not included in this study, nor were those who had a history of no response to neuroleptics.

Haloperidol plasma levels were averaged during fixed- dose treatment and clinical change was measured by the change from baseline on the BPRS psychosis cluster (Thought Disturbance + Hostile Suspiciousness clusters). These data were fit to a theoretical model that proposed the presence of two sigmoidal dose-effect functions, one resulting in a positive treatment response and the other in toxicity or other negative effects as suggested by Teicher and Baldessarini (1985). In this two-component model, the predicted BPRS change score is obtained by subtracting the negative or toxic component from the positive or therapeutic component.

Results

Figure 4–1 shows this two-component model superimposed on a scatter-plot diagram of change in BPRS psychosis factor versus mean plasma haloperidol (multiple $r = .46$, $P < .001$). It appears reasonable to divide the data into the following ranges: < 2 ng/ml (ineffective), 2–5 ng/ml (threshold), 5–12 ng/ml (optimal), and >12 ("toxic"). Mean improvement on the BPRS psychosis factor was significantly greater by t test in the "optimal" versus the "toxic" range ($P = .004$) or the threshold range ($P = .004$) (Table 4–2). Mean improvement in the "optimal" range was roughly twice that in the "threshold" and "toxic" ranges. The standardized effect sizes were both "large" (0.95 and 0.90, respectively).

Reducing Excessive Plasma Levels

Thirteen patients had mean haloperidol plasma levels defined as "excessive" (>12 ng/ml) at the end of the fixed-dose period. Three insisted on leaving the hospital before a dose adjustment was possible. All had become more paranoid (BPRS-P = −3.5, SD 2.5) and two had become extremely

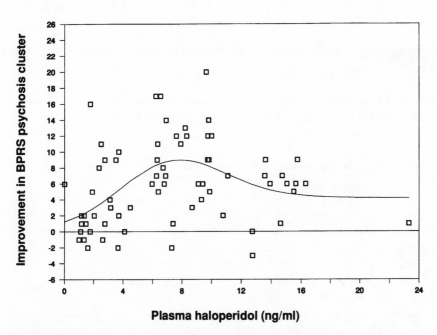

Figure 4–1. Curvilinear relationship between plasma concentration of haloperidol and change in Brief Psychiatric Rating Scale (Overall and Gorham 1962) psychosis factor.

dysphoric. Two patients refused dose reduction. The remaining eight either experienced lesser side effects (in particular a subjective sense of sedation and/or objective akinesia), became less psychotic (5 out of 8), less dysphoric (3 out of 8), and less retarded (8 out 8) when their plasma level was reduced to <12 ng/ml (range = 4.0–10.8 ng/ml, mean = 7.8 ng/ml). No case deteriorated. Table 4–3 summarizes these changes.

Raising Plasma Levels in Relatively Nonresponsive Patients

In eight relatively nonresponsive patients (defined as a global improvement rating of "minimally improved" or less) with plasma levels in the 2–12

Table 4–2. Improvement in four plasma level ranges

| | Range | | | |
	Ineffective <2 ng/ml	Threshold 2–5 ng/ml	Optimal 5.1–12 ng/ml	Suboptimal >12 ng/ml
n	12	14	30	13
Improvement on BPRS psychosis factor (mean ± SD)	2.4 ± 4.9	4.2 ± 4.4	8.8 ± 5.0	4.6 ± 3.7

Note. BPRS = Brief Psychiatric Rating Scale (Overall and Gorham 1962).

Table 4–3. Effect of reducing mean ± SD plasma haloperidol levels

Weeks	Haloperidol (ng/ml)	BPRS-S	BPRS-D	BPRS-P	BPRS-R
1–4	15.0 ± 2.1	5.1 ± 1.6	1.0 ± 4.3	2.4 ± 2.9	− 2.3 ± 3.4
5–8	7.8 ± 2.1	6.4 ± 2.2	2.8 ± 3.8	3.0 ± 3.5	− 0.1 ± 3.8
	t score	2.76	1.82	1.93	5.34
	P value	< .05	NS	< .10	< .01

Note. Ratings are on Brief Psychiatric Rating Scale (BPRS) schizophrenia (S), depression (D), paranoia (P), and retardation (R) factors. Higher change scores mean more improvement; A negative (-) score means deterioration. Change scores relative to baseline (mean ± SD) by paired t test; two-tailed.

ng/ml range, the plasma level was raised above 12 ng/ml (range = 12.9–24 ng/ml, mean = 17.8 ng/ml). Six of eight patients did worse on the global improvement ratings and became more dysphoric. Table 4–4 summarizes the changes.

Discussion

A curvilinear relationship between plasma haloperidol and clinical response was found in these acutely exacerbated patients, most of whom had not taken a neuroleptic for 6 months or more. The upper and lower limits of this proposed therapeutic window were 12 and 5 ng/ml, respectively. When plasma levels in relatively nonresponsive patients were pushed beyond 12 ng/ml (as in routine clinical practice), the patients deteriorated. In particular, they became (relative to their status at the "therapeutic" plasma level) more dysphoric (BPRS Depression Factor −2.6, SD 2.8, $P < .07$); more withdrawn (Withdrawal-Retardation Factor −1.3, SD 2.6, NS); and did not improve in global psychosis ratings (Schizophrenia + Paranoid Factor −0.83, SD 3.4, NS).

Similarly, when patients with plasma levels greater than 12 ng/ml had their plasma levels lowered, they improved (BPRS Schizophrenia +1.25, $P < .05$; Withdrawal Retardation +2.1, $P < .01$). No case deteriorated. Some improved in the sense that they no longer appeared overmedicated in terms of a personal sense of sedation and/or objective akinesia. Three pa-

Table 4–4. Effects of increasing mean ± SD plasma level in relatively nonresponsive patients

Weeks	Haloperidol (ng/ml)	BPRS-S	BPRS-D	BPRS-P	BPRS-R
1–4	7.0 ± 4.0	1.7 ± 2.2	− 1.2 ± 2.7	1.5 ± 2.3	+ 0.3 ± 1.2
5–8	17.8 ± 5.0	2.7 ± 2.0	− 3.8 ± 4.1	− 0.3 ± 2.6	− 1.0 ± 2.2
	t score		2.33		
	P value	NS	.067	NS	NS

Note. Ratings are on Brief Psychiatric Rating Scale (BPRS) schizophrenia (S), depression (D), paranoia (P), and retardation (R) factors. Higher change scores mean more improvement. A negative (−) score means deterioration. Change scores are relative to baseline (mean± SD) by paired t test, two-tailed.

tients with plasma levels greater than 12 ng/ml became globally worse, developed a frantic agitation, and insisted on leaving the hospital before their plasma levels could be lowered (two of these patients had become profoundly depressed). Finally, two patients developed delusions of bodily destruction that disappeared as the plasma level was lowered into the therapeutic range. We, like Quitkin et al. (1975), believe that delusions of bodily destruction can be a psychotic interpretation of neuroleptic toxicity.

We do not mean to imply that patients with plasma levels greater than 12 ng/ml cannot improve relative to their baseline (it is not unusual for schizophrenic patients in the United States to be treated with plasma levels >12 ng/ml) (Reardon et al. 1989). Table 4–5 dichotomizes patients into either improved ("much" or "very much") versus not improved ("minimal improvement," "no change", or "minimally worse.") Five patients were rated "improved" at plasma levels greater than 12 ng/ml.

The division of the data into "ineffective", "threshold", "optimal", and "suboptimal" ranges is by subjective assessment and must be regarded as an approximation. For example, the upper limit of the "optimal" range could well be 10 ng/ml. Clinically, the most important range is the suboptimal or "toxic" (>12 ng/ml) range, which in our study contained only 13 patients. Although plasma level reduction into the 5–12 ng/ml range in 8 of these 13 patients resulted in improved psychosis ratings, the same or greater improvement in psychosis ratings (but not in retardation ratings) could have occurred had these patients been exposed to another 4 weeks on the same suboptimal plasma level. To confirm a "toxic" or suboptimal range, half of the patients in the "toxic" range would need to be randomly assigned to the 5–12 ng/ml range and the other half would need to remain at the toxic

Table 4–5. Global improvement at the end of fixed-dose period

Range	Haloperidol (ng/ml)	Mean level ± SD	Improved (n)	(%)	Not improved (n)	(%)	Ratio (I/NI)
Ineffective	< 2	1.3 ± 0.5	1	9	10	91	0.10
Threshold	2–5	3.2 ± 0.7	6	43	8	57	0.75
Optimal	5–12	8.2 ± 1.6	22	73	8	27	2.75
Suboptimal	> 12	15.2 ± 2.7	5	39	8	62	0.63

Note. "Improved" (I) = "very much" or "much improved"; "Not improved" (NI) = "minimal improvement," "no change," or "minimally worse" on the Clinical Global Impression (CGI) Scale (National Institute of Mental Health 1985). Total $N = 68$; $\chi^2 = 10.75$, df = 3, $P = .013$.

level range. Therefore, a clear decrease in antipsychotic effect at doses of haloperidol greater than 12 ng/ml has not been demonstrated.

Because the correlation between dose and plasma level for haloperidol is rather high (r = .76) in this and other studies, a plasma level usually does not add much additional information when the clinician already knows the dose. On a dose of 10–15 mg/day nearly all patients would be in the therapeutic window (Table 4–6). Recent work from the Karolinska Institute (Llerena et al. 1992) however, indicates that about 7% of Caucasians may be at risk of developing side effects as the result of aberrantly high plasma haloperidol levels (7% of Caucasians have a decreased capacity to hydroxylate debrisoquine and in the study by Llerena et al. [1992], the patients with poor debrisoquine metabolization eliminated a 4-g haloperidol dose more slowly than patients who metabolize debrisoquine normally. Furthermore, the patients who metabolized debrisoquine poorly developed severe extrapyramidal symptoms [EPS]).

Does knowledge of plasma level improve prediction of outcome over and above knowledge of dose? Using a more conventional method of evaluating a curvilinear relationship (a curvilinear [quadratic] function of plasma level fits the data better than a quadratic function of dose [multiple r plasma = .40, df = 2,66, P = .003; multiple r dose = .28, df = 2,66, P = .07]) and a stepwise multiple regression analysis indicated that plasma level produces a significant increment in the multiple r values (F = 3.75, df = 2,64, P = .03). Thus plasma level is the more powerful predictor of outcome.

Consequently, it would seem prudent to consider dose reduction in any nonresponsive patient with a plasma level greater than 12 ng/ml. Similarly, it may also be prudent to measure plasma haloperidol in responsive pa-

Table 4–6. Dose versus plasma level of haloperidol

	Dose		
	5 mg/day (n = 21)	10 mg/day (n = 31)	20 mg/day (n = 17)
Mean ± SD plasma haloperidol (ng/ml)	2.2 ± .9	7.7 ± 3.2	12.8 ± 4.0
Range	1.0 – 4.1	0 – 15.6	7.6 – 23.3
SEM	0.2	0.6	1.0

Note. For each patient weekly plasma levels were averaged. Haloperidol versus dose, r = .78, P < .0001.

tients who are on a high dose. If the plasma haloperidol is greater than 12 ng/ml, a trial of dose reduction may be indicated. Lastly, plasma haloperidol level measurements may be most informative with respect to drug interactions. For example, carbamazepine is known to reduce plasma haloperidol levels by 50% or more through microsomal enzyme induction (Ereshefsky et al. 1984; Jann et al. 1985; Fast et al. 1986) and other drug interactions are likely to be discovered.

The reason why patients tend not to do as well at plasma levels greater than 12 ng/ml is unknown. It is unclear whether efficacy is lost above a certain plasma level or whether adverse effects diminish therapeutic response. Our clinical sense indicates that the latter is true, but there was no relationship in our study between plasma haloperidol level and objectively rated akinesia or akathisia. However when side effects were rated on the Clinical Global Impression (CGI) Scale (National Institute of Mental Health 1985), there was a powerful relationship between plasma haloperidol and what the patient experienced as "disabling side effects" (defined as "side effects that significantly interfered with patient's functioning" or "side effects that outweighed therapeutic effects"). Figure 4–2 shows the relationship between plasma haloperidol and "disabling side effects" significant at the $P = .0002$ level by using logistic regression.

Disabling side effect data were obtained by the senior investigator (TVP) during semistructured interviews in which side effects were specifically inquired about. Thus if a patient stated that a certain amount of drowsiness, restlessness, jitteriness, or a feeling of being "slowed down" was unbearable to him, the side effect would be listed as "outweighing therapeutic effects" even though, objectively, the patient might not have appeared drowsy, slowed down, or akathesic. If the patient indicated that the side effects would interfere with functioning outside of the hospital, the side effect was listed as "significantly interferes with patient's functioning." Using these ratings, 69% of the patients who had plasma haloperidol ranges between 12 and 23 ng/ml experienced "disabling side effects."

These findings concur with McEvoy et al. (1991), who reported substantial dose-related increases in bradykinesia (effect size, 1.39) and akathisia (effect size, 1.61) as reported by the patient and in subjective states such as "sluggish," "anxious," "dysphoric," and "feels bad" (effect sizes ranged from 0.35 to 0.68). These increases occurred with haloperidol at a mean dose of 11.6 ± 4.7 mg/day, which should result in haloperidol plasma levels comparable with the doses in our study. Also in McEvoy's study (1991), the amount of bradykinesia and akathisia reported by patients was about twice the amount of bradykinesia and akathisia observed by the investigators.

Disabling side effects were correlated with ratings of akinesia (r = .40, P = .001), akathisia (r = .35, P = .003) and akathisia plus akinesia (r = .48, P = .0001). The objective ratings of akathisia and akinesia were mild or very mild in 37% of patients; ratings as low as these probably would be dismissed in many other settings. Weiden (1985) showed that akathisia was markedly underdiagnosed in most clinical settings. The relationship between plasma haloperidol levels and side effects, as experienced by the patient, suggests that side effects—at least in acutely exacerbated patients—contribute to the poorer clinical response at plasma levels greater than 12 ng/ml.

Our proposed range of 5 to 12 ng/ml may not apply to the more chronic, treatment-refractory patient. Certainly many such patients are stabilized at plasma levels of haloperidol much greater than 12 ng/ml (Van Putten et al. 1985). The fact that such patients, to various degrees, can tolerate such high levels does not, however, mean that this is their optimal plasma level. Furthermore, the higher plasma levels in some treatment-refractory patients are really used for "chemical restraint" or result from the compulsion to "do something."

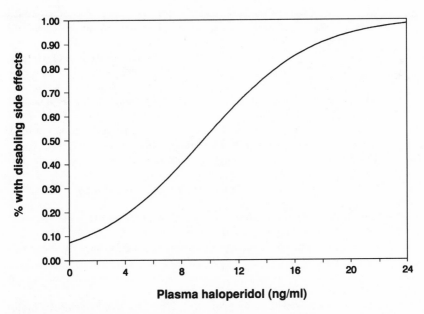

Figure 4–2. Disabling side effects and plasma halperidol. Logistic regression model, N = 68, χ^2 = 13.5, P = .0002.

References

American Psychiatric Association: Diagnostic and Statistical Manual of Mental Disorders, 3rd Edition. Washington, DC, American Psychiatric Association, 1980

Bigelow LB, Kirch DG, Korpi BT, et al: Absence of relationship of serum haloperidol concentration and clinical response in chronic schizophrenia: a fixed-dose study. Psychopharmacol Bull 21:66–68, 1985

Bleeker JAC, Dingemans PM, Frohn-De Winder ML: Plasma level and effect of low-dose haloperidol in acute psychosis. Psychopharmacol Bull 20:317–319, 1984.

Coryell W, Kelly M, Perry PJ, et al: Haloperidol plasma levels and acute clinical change in schizophrenia. J Clin Psychopharmacol 10:397–402, 1990

Ereshefsky L, Davis CM, Harrington CA: Haloperidol and reduced haloperidol plasma levels in selected schizophrenic patients. J Clin Psychopharmacol 4:138–142, 1984

Fast DK, Jones BD, Kusalic M, et al: Effect of carbamazepine on neuroleptic plasma level and efficacy (letter). Am J Psychiatry 143:117–118, 1986

Itoh H, Yagi G, Fuji Y, et al: The relationship between haloperidol blood levels and clinical responses. Prog Neuropsychopharmacol Biol Psychiatry 8:285–292, 1984

Jann MW, Ereshefsky L, Saklad SR: Effects of carbamazepine on plasma haloperidol levels. J Clin Psychopharmacol 5:106–109, 1985

Linkowski P, Hubain P, von Frenckell R, et al: Haloperidol plasma levels and clinical response in paranoid schizophrenics. Eur Arch Psychiatry Neurol Sci 234:231–236, 1984

Llerena A, Dahl ML, Ekgvist B, et al: Genetic factors in the metabolism of haloperidol. Clin Neuropharmacol (suppl) 15: 84A–85A, 1992

McEvoy JP, Hogarty GE, Steingard S: Optimal dose of neuroleptic in acute schizophrenia: a controlled study of the neuroleptic threshold and higher haloperidol dose. Arch Gen Psychiatry 48:739–745, 1991

Mavroidis ML, Kanter DR, Hirschozitz J, et al: Clinical response and plasma haloperidol levels in schizophrenia. Psychopharmacology 81:354–356, 1983

National Institute of Mental Health: CGI (Clinical Global Impression) Scale. Psychopharmacol Bull 21:839–843, 1985

Overall JE, Gorham DR: The Brief Psychiatric Rating Scale. Psychol Rep 10:799–812, 1962

Potkin SG, Shen Y, Zhou D, et al: Does a therapeutic window for plasma haloperidol exist? Preliminary Chinese data. Psychopharmacol Bull 21:59–61, 1985

Quitkin F, Rifkin A, Klein DF: Very high dosage vs standard dosage fluphenazine in schizophrenia. Arch Gen Psychiatry 32:1276–1281, 1975

Reardon GT, Rifkin A, Schwartz A, et al: Changing patterns of neuroleptic dosage over a decade. Am J Psychiatry 146:726–729, 1989

Rimon R, Averbuch I, Rozick P, et al: Serum and CSF levels of haloperidol by radioimmunoassay and radioreceptor assay during high-dose therapy of resistant schizophrenic patients. Psychopharmacology 73:197–199, 1981

Santos JL, Cabranes JA, Almoguera I: Clinical implications of determination of plasma haloperidol levels. Acta Psychiatr Scand 79:348–354, 1989

Simpson GM, Angus JWG: A rating scale for extrapyramidal side effects. Acta Psychiatr Scand Suppl 212:11–19, 1970

Smith RC, Baumgartner R, Misra CH: Haloperidol, plasma levels and prolactin response as predictors of clinical improvement in schizophrenia: chemical vs. radioreceptor plasma level assay. Arch Gen Psychiatry 41:1044–1049, 1984

Teicher MH, Baldessarini RJ: Selection of neuroleptic dosage. Arch Gen Psychiatry 42:636–637, 1985

Van Putten T, Marder SR, May PRA, et al: Plasma levels of haloperidol and clinical response. Psychopharmacol Bull 21:69–72, 1985

Van Putten T, Marder SR, Mintz J: A controlled dose comparison of haloperidol in newly admitted schizophrenic patients. Arch Gen Psychiatry 47:754–758, 1990

Volavka J, Cooper TB, Meisner M, et al: Haloperidol blood levels and effects in schizophrenia and schizoaffective disorder: a progress report. Psychopharmacol Bull 26:13–17, 1990

Weiden P: Akathisia from prochlorperazine (letter). JAMA 253:635, 1985

Wistedt B, Johanidesz G, Omerhodzic M, et al: Plasma haloperidol levels and clinical response in acute schizophrenia. Nord Psychiatr Tidsskr 1:9–13, 1984

CHAPTER 5

Haloperidol Plasma Levels and Initial Response to Neuroleptic Treatment

John M. Davis, M.D.
Stephen E. Ericksen, M.D.
Stephen Hurt, Ph.D.
Sidney S. Chang, M.D.
Javaid I. Javaid, Ph.D.
Haroutune Dekirmenjian, Ph.D.
Regina Casper, M.D.

I n naturalistic studies in the late 1960s, Curry and colleagues (1968, 1970a, 1970b) investigated the relationship between plasma chlorpromazine levels and clinical response. The best clinical response was found with moderate chlorpromazine levels. Patients who had low plasma chlorpromazine levels showed poorer clinical response with minimal side effects. Extremely high chlorpromazine plasma levels were also associated with poor clinical response but with a moderate level of side effects. We suggest that an inverted U-shaped relationship exists between therapeutic response and plasma levels.

✦ In patients who metabolize chlorpromazine rapidly with the consequent low plasma levels, insufficient drug reaches the brain to produce neither a therapeutic effect nor side effects.
✦ In patients who metabolize chlorpromazine at a moderate rate and have moderate plasma levels, a good therapeutic response occurs with only mild side effects.
✦ In patients with high plasma chlorpromazine levels because of a defect

in metabolism, excessive side effects may interfere with therapeutic response, and excessive sedation and extrapyramidal side effects (EPS) such as akathisia might interfere with the beneficial effect of the drug in some sense.

In addition, Curry and colleagues (1968, 1970a,b) originally suggested that chlorpromazine might lose its efficacy at high plasma levels. There may be two meanings to the upper end of the therapeutic window: excessive side effects and possible loss of efficacy.

It should be readily apparent that uncontrolled observations do not constitute proof of an inverted U-shaped relationship between therapeutic response and plasma levels. Clinicians increase a patient's dose when the patient fails to show a clinical response, and with an increase in dose, the patient will have a higher plasma level. Thus the upper end of the therapeutic window is artifactual in this context. Because flexible-dose studies are methodologically flawed, one cannot make valid conclusions about the relationship of plasma levels to efficacy from this design, i.e., the dose determines plasma level, but the dose, in turn, is determined by the clinician's judgment based on the patient's clinical state.

In a therapeutic trial, it is necessary to study patients who have florid illness and, therefore, have the capacity to show a substantial degree of therapeutic improvement, and for the investigator to accurately quantitate degrees of improvement. Chronic, relatively stabilized "end-stage," long-term hospitalized patients are not valid for plasma level-efficacy studies because the drugs have produced all the effects of which they are capable. It is also important to distinguish rate of improvement from maximal improvement possible. We expect the former to be related to blood levels and the latter to correlate with the underlying prognosis of the patient. The highest rate of drug-induced improvement is in the first week of treatment; after a few weeks of treatment the rate of improvement decreases gradually because it abuts on the capacity of the patient to improve. Therefore, the rate of improvement in the first week or two is the most valued measure of improvement induced by the drug.

In summary, in our judgment, the two important methodological requirements for a sound study are: 1) floridly ill patients who would be expected to show good improvement, and 2) a fixed-dose strategy. By fixed dose, we mean a dose with either all patients assigned to one fixed dose or the random assignment of patients to a low and high fixed dose (or even to three or four different doses). This assigned predetermined dose is then followed throughout the length of the trial.

Methods

Study patients were 35 acutely decompensated schizophrenic patients (diagnosed according to the Research Diagnostic Criteria [RDC; Spitzer et al. 1978]) who had consecutive voluntary admissions to a research ward at the Illinois State Psychiatric Institute, who were in good physical health, and were between 18 and 43 years old. After signing an informed consent, patients were randomly assigned to receive either: 1) a high loading dose, or 2) a standard-dose treatment by the hospital pharmacist. All had clear signs of schizophrenia that persisted beyond an initial 7- to 18-day drug-free washout period. The patients in each treatment group were similar in age, age at onset of illness, number of previous hospitalizations, length of present hospitalization, sex distribution, subtype diagnosis, and mean number of family members with a history of psychiatric disorders.

High loading-dose patients received haloperidol 60 mg/day im in six divided doses of 10 mg for the first 5 days of treatment plus placebo tablets. They were then switched to oral haloperidol at the following dosages: 45 mg/day po for 2 days, 30 mg/day po for 2 days, 20 mg/day po for 3 days, and finally 15 mg/day po for the final week of study. Patients assigned to the standard-dose schedule received 15 mg/day po for the full 3 weeks plus placebo injections. A double-blind technique was used; both groups received exactly the same number of injections and tablets.

The Brief Psychiatric Rating Scale (BPRS; Overall and Gorham 1962) and the Clinical Global Impression Scale (CGI; National Institute of Mental Health 1985) were used to rate each patient during the baseline period and five times during the 3 weeks of treatment. The rating team consisted of a staff psychiatrist, a senior psychiatric resident, and a psychiatric social worker. Double-blind methodology was used with strict blind maintenance for plasma levels and group assignment. "Responder" status was classified by a medial split of percent of change of BPRS or CGI at week 2. Benztropine mesylate (Cogentin) in appropriate parenteral and/or oral doses was used to manage EPS. Haloperidol (Haldol) plasma levels were determined by gas chromatography by using a slightly modified method of Javaid et al. (1979).

The patients improved very rapidly in the first week, with improvement continuing in the second or third week but at a less rapid rate. The average plasma level during the first 2 weeks of treatment was calculated. It was recognized that patients were not at steady-state levels in the first week and that the dose was decreasing in the second week. The observed plasma levels cannot be considered to reflect steady-state levels, but plasma levels measured before a steady state was achieved would be expected to correlate reasonably well with plasma levels after steady state was achieved if a constant fixed loading dose was used for the entire study. Doses were fixed at the previously defined levels and not altered clinically.

Results

When plasma levels were divided into three groups (low, < 5 ng/ml; moderate, 5–21 ng/ml; high, 22 ng/ml or more), we found an inverted U-shaped relationship between average plasma haloperidol levels during the first 2 weeks of treatment and clinical response as assessed by both the CGI and the BPRS. Most of the nonresponsive patients on both CGI and BPRS had either low or high plasma levels (Table 5–1). A 2×3 χ^2 was statistically significant. Patients receiving a high dose had higher plasma levels than those receiving a standard dose, but there was a substantial degree of variability in plasma levels between both groups with overlap of the plasma levels between the high dose and the standard dose.

Because we predicted that the low and high plasma level groups would have a better response than the group with plasma levels in the therapeutic window, we tested the data with an analysis of variance using a Helmert contrast that tested the latter group against the combined low and high groups (which we predicted to be significant) and the low versus high group (which we predicted not to be significant). The overall F test was significant for the CGI ($F = 3.91$, df = 1, $P = .03$), and the first Helmert con-

Table 5–1. Clinical response at varying plasma levels of haloperidol

	CGI				BPRS			
	NR		R		NR		R	
Plasma level	(n)	($\%$)	(n)	($\%$)	(n)	($\%$)	(n)	($\%$)
Low	5	71	2	29	3	43	4	57
Medium	5	26	14	74	6	32	13	68
High	7	78	2	22	8	89	1	11

Note. CGI = Clinical Global Impression Scale (National Institute of Mental Health 1985); BPRS = Brief Psychiatric Rating Scale (Overall and Gorham 1962); NR = patients who did not respond ("nonresponders"); R = patients who did respond ("responders"). For CGI, $\chi^2 = 8.3$, df = 2, $P = .016$. For BPRS, χ^2 8.14, df = 2, $P = .017$.

trast (inside versus outside the therapeutic window) yielded $t = 2.59$, df = 1, $P = .01$ and the second Helmert contrast yielded $t = .8$, $P = $ NS. The overall F test for the BPRS was significant ($F = 5.11$, df = 1, $P = .01$), and the first Helmert contrast yielded $t = 2.11$, $P = .01$ and the second Helmert contrast yielded $t = 2.2$, $P = .04$, with less improvement in those with a high plasma level. The Mean Percent Change scores for CGI and BPRS for the low, middle (within window), and high group were −23%, −39%, −14% and −37%, −39%, −19%, respectively.

Discussion

Empirically, we found a curvilinear relationship between plasma levels and clinical response, with patients having a poor response also having either low or high plasma levels; however the order of magnitude of the curvilinear response was not that impressive statistically. Both the evidence for a therapeutic window and the variable of this correlation we found in our data are consistent with that expected based on other data, much of which is summarized in this book. We emphasize that the plasma levels were not obtained during steady state and cannot be compared in their exact absolute amounts with true steady-state levels. It is expected that when steady state was reached, the same rank ordering of plasma levels would be obtained, but the reader should be aware that this is a rank-ordering judgment based on nonsteady-state values and that only an interpolation for comparison with steady-state studies is being made. Obviously, only studies that used a low dose are most appropriate for defining the low threshold plasma level (the low end of the therapeutic window), and we only had seven patients with low plasma levels which was clearly a small number with its obvious limitations.

Most fixed-dose studies for floridly ill patients found poor clinical response at low plasma levels and good clinical response at moderate plasma levels. In some studies, when high plasma levels are reached, there was poor clinical response at high plasma levels.

In many cases, as in our study, the statistical significance of the relationship was weak, just near the 5% level of statistical significance. Our study found a great deal of scatter in the data and it is clear that there is not a one-to-one relationship between plasma level and therapeutic efficacy. There are two separate questions to be determined. The first is determination of the threshold plasma level. It is possible that superimposed on the considerable variability in the data is a threshold plasma level of haloperidol in the region of 5 ng/ml. It is of interest that this is similar to the threshold plasma level found by other investigators. Obviously, if a study focuses on the upper end of the therapeutic window and the total group of patients receives only high doses, no patients may have an inadequate dose and be below the threshold. Therefore, any such study is nonrelevant to finding the therapeutic threshold plasma level. We would like to add a methodological caveat here. Investigators can perform studies and arbitrarily define the lower end of the therapeutic window, or for that matter, an upper end of the therapeutic window, choosing a particularly fortunate cutoff point, and consequently, these data are a best-case scenario. If we review multiple studies and choose these arbitrarily defined cutoff points in each study, this method carries with it the constant error statistically associated with letting the data define the optimal cutoff point to define a given relationship. It is more appropriate to examine the first few studies to see what a reasonable cutoff point is and then test this cutoff point in a prospective study. Small studies are important in helping us to find a reasonable point to define the lower end of the therapeutic window, or more precisely, the lower threshold plasma level. This proposed cutoff point must be tested in large studies for that purpose, with sufficient statistical power to provide an answer.

The same considerations apply to testing whether there is an upper end of the therapeutic window. In that situation we would expect more variability and also expect that the upper end would be rather fuzzy. We would expect that those patients who are particularly vulnerable to a particular side effect (e.g., excessive sedation and akathisia) would do especially poorly.

Because we hypothesize that there is a threshold plasma level, a linear correlation does not capture the data as exactly as a sigmoidal curve does. We are forced to think of thresholds as a discontinuous variable. Defining both the upper and lower ends of the therapeutic window is much more problematical. Fitting data to a quadratic function when unequal numbers of patients are at each end of the therapeutic window is a massive departure from reasonable assumptions and is essentially valueless under most circumstances. In the absence of an appropriate statistical model, we are dependent on cutoff points, but the above qualification must be kept in mind.

A number of studies have provided evidence relevant to the upper end of the therapeutic window. Here, the study must have patients with normal plasma levels and unusually high plasma levels to be pertinent. Here the data is more variable, because we find a hint of an upper end of the therapeutic window. We hasten to qualify that not all investigators do, and this must be regarded as tentative.

References

Curry SH, Davis JM, Janowsky D, et al: Intrapatient variation in physiological availability of chlorpromazine as a complicating factor in correlation studies of drug metabolism and clinical effect, in The Present Status of Psychotropic Drugs, Vol 6. Amsterdam, Excerpta Medica Foundation, 1968, pp 72–76

Curry SH, Janowsky DS, Davis JM, et al: Factors affecting chlorpromazine plasma levels in psychiatric patients. Arch Gen Psychiatry 22:209–215, 1970a

Curry SH, Marshall JHL, Davis JM, et al: Chlorpromazine plasma levels and effects. Arch Gen Psychiatry 22:289–296, 1970b

Javaid JI, Dekirmenjian H, Liskevyah V, et al. Determination of butaperazine in biological fluids by gas chromatography using nitrogen specific detection system. J Chromatogr Sci 17:666–670, 1979

National Institute of Mental Health: CGI (Clinical Global Impression) Scale. Psychopharmacol Bull 21:839–843, 1985

Overall JE, Gorham DR: The Brief Psychiatric Rating Scale. Psychol Rep 10:799–812, 1962

Spitzer RL, Endicott J, Robins E: Research Diagnostic Criteria: rationale and reliability. Arch Gen Psychiatry 35:773–782, 1978

CHAPTER 6

Clinical Use of Clozapine Plasma Concentrations

Paul J. Perry, Ph.D.
Del D. Miller, Pharm.D., M.D.

C lozapine, a dibenzodiazepine, is the first and only atypical antipsy-chotic approved for use in the United States. It represents the first major new treatment for schizophrenia in over 20 years. Its thera-peutic efficacy is hypothesized to result from either dopamine (D) block-ade alone or a combination of serotonin and dopamine blockade. The drug has a more balanced pharmacologic antagonism of both subtype 1 (D_1) and subtype 2 (D_2) receptors and greater inhibition of D_1 receptor-coupled adenylate cyclase than the phenothiazine, thioxanthene, or butyrophenone neuroleptics. Thus the drug is regarded as an atypical neu-roleptic (Meltzer et al. 1989).

Studies of acute schizophrenia have shown clozapine to be at least as effective, and often more effective, than standard antipsychotics (Guirguis et al. 1977; Shopsin et al. 1979). Clozapine is now considered to be more effective than other neuroleptics in the treatment of traditional neurolep-tic-resistant schizophrenic patients. Kane et al. (1988) found that 38 (30%) treatment-resistant chronic schizophrenic patients improved when treated with clozapine, compared with 5 (4%) patients who improved with chlor-promazine. In the clozapine-treated group, improvement was seen in both positive and negative symptoms of schizophrenia.

Initial European studies found either a weak correlation or no correla-tion between clinical response and clozapine plasma concentrations.

From the Mental Health Research Center—Major Psychoses, funded in part by NIMH Grant 5 P50-MH43271.

Ackenheil et al. (1976) studied 26 schizophrenic or schizoaffective patients. They were treated with a nonfixed dose of clozapine that varied from 100–600 mg/day for 30 days. The investigators were unable to demonstrate a relationship between clozapine plasma concentrations and symptoms evaluated with the Association for Methodology and Documentation in Psychiatry (AMDP) rating system (Guy and Ban 1982). Two years later, the same group (Brau et al. 1978) again examined the relationship between clozapine and therapeutic response in 32 patients with a paranoid-hallucinating syndrome. Because patients were given doses "according to clinical demands," it was assumed that a fixed dose of drug was not used during the 30-day trial. Only on the third day of treatment were the investigators able to observe a significant relationship between plasma concentrations and improvement. The patients' paranoid and manic symptoms demonstrated significant improvement ($P < .01$). Ackenheil (1989) described 32 psychiatric patients treated with variable doses of clozapine for 30 days. The patients had ICD-9 diagnoses that included schizophrenia ($n = 12$), schizoaffective disorder ($n = 8$), mania ($n = 3$), and schizophreniform disorder ($n = 9$). The daily dose ranged from 100–875 mg/day. Clozapine plasma concentrations and the clinical outcome variables measured with the AMDP rating system correlated weakly only on the first day of treatment. Similar to the previous studies, the obvious problem with the design was that the dose was not fixed, thereby invalidating any positive findings.

In another study, Thorup and Fog (1977) treated 11 hospitalized male chronic schizophrenic patients with a fixed dose of clozapine. The dose ranged from 200–600 mg/day for a minimum of 12 weeks. Although the patients were on fixed doses throughout the study period, individual doses were dictated by the patient's previous response, which obviously biased the results. The authors reported that the plasma concentrations appeared to have no correlation with clinical effect. They did not describe in their methodology how they measured clinical effect. Thus a total of four studies from two clinical centers suggested no relationship was apparent between clozapine plasma concentrations and therapeutic response.

Perry et al. (1991a) described a fixed-dose study of clozapine in treatment-refractory schizophrenic patients. Patients met DSM-III-R criteria (American Psychiatric Association 1987) for a diagnosis of schizophrenia as determined by a consensus of two psychiatrists. All patients were previously treated with at least three 6-week neuroleptic courses representing at least two chemically dissimilar phenothiazine or butyrophenone classes with a does of chlorpromazine (750 mg/day or its equivalent) without substantial relief of symptoms within the past 5 years. The baseline 18-item anchored Brief Psychiatric Rating Scale (BPRS; Overall and Gorham 1962) score exceeded 40 in all patients. No depot neuroleptics were used during the preceding 6 weeks. Clozapine was then initiated at a dose of 50 mg/day, and increased by 50 mg/day when tolerated by the patient to the maximum tolerable dose or a peak dose of 400 mg/day. The patients were maintained on this dose of clozapine for a 4-week period. On the day of admission and after each week of fixed-dose therapy, patients were rated using the BPRS, the Scale for Assessment of Positive Symptoms (SAPS; Andreasen 1984), and the Scale for Assessment of Negative Symptoms (SANS; Andreasen 1982, 1983). Following clozapine titration, blood samples were drawn for the clozapine essay at the same time the rating scales were administered.

Twenty-nine patients completed the 4-week, fixed-dose clozapine trial. Subjects received a mean clozapine dose of 384 ± 42 mg/day, equivalent to 4.9 ± 1.0 mg/kg body weight per day. It required 10.5 ± 3.3 days (range = 7–24 days) for the patients to be titrated to their maximum tolerable dose. Of the patients who improved on clozapine, there was no difference in the dose between the "responders" (4.6 ± 1.0 mg/kg body weight per day) and the "nonresponders" (5.2 ± 1.1 mg/kg body weight per day). Twenty-four of 29 patients received 400 mg/day, although 5 patients were unable to tolerate the high dose. The limiting adverse effect in all five patients was daytime sedation. Because there were no statistical intraindividual differences among the four weekly clozapine and desmethyclozapine concentrations, the mean clozapine concentration was used to characterize each patient. The mean clozapine and norclozapine values were 374 ± 233 and 116 ± 65 ng/ml, respectively. Table 6–1 summarizes the clozapine plasma concentration and response data for the 29 patients.

Receiver Operating Characteristic Curves

The optimal split for the clozapine concentrations was estimated by drawing Receiver Operating Characteristic (ROC) curves (Mossman and Somoza 1991). To construct a ROC curve, the percentages of responsive patients in the presence of a signal ("true positive responders," i.e., responsive patients at a particular clozapine plasma concentration) are plotted on the y-axis against the percentage of nonresponsive patients in the absence of the signal ("false positive responders," i.e., nonresponsive patients at a particular clozapine plasma concentration) on the x-axis. Unlike the original analysis of the data (Perry et al. 1991a), in the ROC curves presented

Table 6–1. Clozapine plasma concentrations and response according to BPRS, SAPS, SANS, and SAPS/SANS overall ratings

Clozapine (ng/ml)	Total clozapine (ng/ml)	BPRS	SAPS	SANS	SAPS + SANS
84	120	NR	NR	NR	NR
100	125	R	R	R	R
122	148	R	R	R	R
128	162	NR	R	NR	NR
200	283	NR	NR	NR	NR
201	291	NR	NR	NR	NR
206	265	NR	NR	NR	NR
213	263	R	R	R	R
213	360	NR	NR	NR	NR
229	295	NR	NR	NR	NR
260	359	R	R	R	R
273	362	NR	NR	NR	NR
280	367	NR	R	NR	NR
283	408	NR	R	R	R
289	385	NR	NR	NR	NR
304	400	NR	NR	NR	NR
307	411	NR	NR	NR	NR
322	418	NR	NR	NR	NR
397	509	R	NR	NR	NR
504	609	R	R	R	R
520	666	R	R	R	R
527	717	R	R	NR	R
544	770	R	R	R	R
549	694	NR	NR	NR	NR
573	779	R	R	R	R
662	804	NR	R	R	R
687	850	R	R	R	R
782	1,026	NR	R	R	R
1,088	1,361	NR	NR	NR	NR

Note. BPRS = Brief Psychiatric Rating Scale (Overall and Gorham 1962); SAPS = Scale for the Assessment of Positive Symptoms (Andreasen 1984); SANS = Scale for the Assessment of Negative Symptoms (Andreasen 1983); NR = subject did not respond to treatment ("nonresponder"); R = subject did respond to treatment ("responder").

in this chapter each data point is graphed separately. In the original data, clozapine plasma concentration ranges were graphed, rather than each point separately. The present figurative representation of the data resulted in a more precise identification of the point of maximum sensitivity and specificity. Commonly, ROC curves do not have each point graphed separately but use ranges, as was originally done. The optimum predictive clozapine plasma concentration on a ROC curve for the following data is located at the point on the curve closest to the y-axis (true positive responders) and furthest from the x-axis (false positive responders). Often this point is less than obvious when the data are visually inspected. Thus the optimum sensitivity point on the graph is that point that has the largest difference when the false positive responders value (x) is subtracted from true positive responders value (y). This point identifies the clozapine concentration that maximizes sensitivity for the drug concentration response marker. The identification of an optimum cutoff point results in the data being practically divided into four categories or rates: true positives, false positives, true negatives, and false negatives. These four rates are the same as those yielded by the 2×2 matrix of a contingency table constructed for a χ^2 analysis. The sensitivity (true positive rate, i.e., ++ cell) and specificity (true negative rate, i.e., – – cell) for the cut-point is then determined by performing a χ^2 analysis to determine if the distribution is significantly different among the four cells.

Brief Psychiatric Rating Scale Response

The BPRS scores of the patients were categorized as "responders" or "nonresponders" according to the criteria of Kane et al. (1988). Improvement or response was defined as an increase of at least 20% in the total BPRS score from baseline to the end of week 4 of a fixed-dose regimen and a final BPRS score of 34 or less. Eleven of the 29 patients (38%) were classified as responders using the above criteria. There were no statistically significant differences between the age, sex distribution, duration of illness, dose, mean clozapine concentration, or norclozapine concentration of the responders and nonresponders. However, the nonresponders did have significantly higher BPRS scores than the responders. To assess the significance of this issue, a multiple linear regression analysis was performed. The dependent variable was the week-4 BPRS score and the independent variables were mean clozapine concentration, mean norclozapine concentration, and baseline BPRS score. The analysis revealed a statistically significant correlation only between the baseline BPRS score and the week-4 BPRS score. However, when a "nonresponder" with a mean steady-state clozapine concentration greater than three standard deviations above the mean (1,088 ng/ml) was removed from the data set, the clozapine variable as well as the baseline BPRS score variable reached significance. Thus based on this initial review of the data, a linear relationship was assumed between clozapine concentrations and change in the BPRS scores (Perry et al. 1991b).

Each patient's BPRS scores were broken down into three symptom factors based on Guy et al.'s (1974) 5-factor Varimax solution of the 18-item BPRS. The anergia factor, the thought disturbance factor, and the interpersonal disturbance factor were used in the analyses. The anergia factor was used as an estimate of the negative symptom response to clozapine. The thought- and interpersonal-disturbance factors were used as indices of the positive symptom response to clozapine. At baseline, the anergia scores of nonresponder's were greater than those of the responders although there was no difference in the other two factor scores. Both the responders and nonresponders showed significant decreases in all three factor scores over their period of clozapine treatment. However, at week 4 scores of the responders were significantly lower for anergia, thought disturbance, and interpersonal disturbance.

Receiver Operating Characteristic Curves and Clozapine Concentration's Sensitivity and Specificity

ROC curves for the clozapine and total clozapine (clozapine + norclozapine) data sets are presented in Figures 6–1 and 6–2. As illustrated in Figure 6–1, a clozapine plasma concentration of 397 ng/ml or greater was the most sensitive cutoff point that differentiated the responders from the nonresponders. As illustrated in Figure 6–2, a total clozapine (clozapine + norclozapine) plasma concentration of at least 509 ng/ml was the obvious cutoff point.

BPRS Response

Clozapine concentrations of 397 ng/ml or higher defined a group of 11 patients that included 7 (64%) of the 11 patients who responded to the drug. Total clozapine concentrations of 509 ng/ml or higher also defined the same group of 11 patients. Thus both drug concentrations produced the same degree of sensitivity. Additionally, both drug concentrations were able to produce the same degree of specificity. Clozapine concentrations of less than 397 ng/ml and total concentrations of less than 509 ng/ml predicted no response in 78% (14 of 18) of the patients. Further, χ^2 analyses on the data found the differences between the responders and non-responders at these particular concentrations significant ($\chi^2 = 4.974$, df = 1, $P = .03$).

SAPS and SANS Response

These two scales were designed to measure more specifically positive and negative symptoms. The SAPS and SANS rating scales were used to deter-

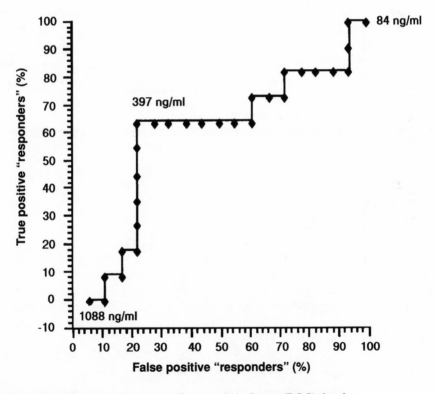

Figure 6–1. Receiver Operating Characteristic Curve (ROC) for the relationship between Brief Psychiatric Rating Scale (BPRS; Overall and Gorham 1962) scores and clozapine plasma concentrations ranging from 84 to 1,088 ng/ml. True positive "responders," $n = 11$; false positive "responders," $n = 18$.

mine if there was a minimum effective clozapine plasma concentration that was required for improvement. The scales would also demonstrate if different concentrations of drug were necessary to produce improvement in positive and negative symptoms and whether the improvements were interrelated or independent. Improvement in positive symptoms was defined as a 20% decrease in the sum of the four global items on the SAPS and a final score of 8. Improvement in negative symptoms was defined as a 20% decrease in the sum of the five global items on the SANS and a final score of 10. Overall improvement was defined as a 20% decrease in the sum of the nine global items on the SAPS and SANS and a final score of 20. Fifteen subjects (52%) showed improvement in positive symptoms. Twelve subjects (41%) showed improvement in negative symptoms. All 12 of the patients who showed improvement in negative symptoms also had improve-

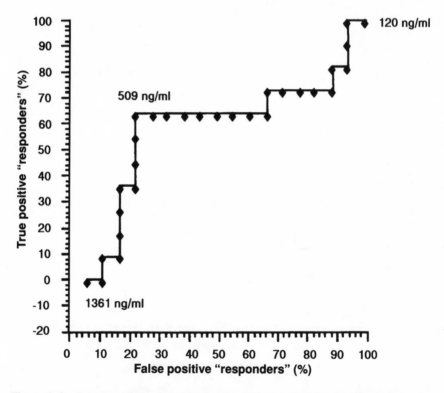

Figure 6–2. Receiver Operating Characteristic Curve (ROC) for the relationship between Brief Psychiatric Rating Scale (BPRS; Overall and Gorham 1962) scores and total clozapine plasma concentrations ranging from 120 to 1361 ng/ml. True positive "responders," $n = 11$; false positive "responders," $n = 18$.

ment in positive symptoms and overall improvement. There was one additional patient that did not show improvement in negative symptoms but was categorized as being improved overall. Thirteen (45%) patients demonstrated overall improvement on the total global scores of the SAPS and SANS.

As illustrated in Figures 6–3, 6–4, and 6–5, a threshold clozapine plasma concentration of 504 ng/ml or more was required for improvement of the positive and negative symptoms as well as overall improvement. For total clozapine (clozapine + norclozapine), a concentration of 609 ng/ml or more produced identical improvement findings.

Clozapine plasma concentrations of 504 ng/ml or more demonstrated a sensitivity of 80% and a specificity of 63% for improvement in positive

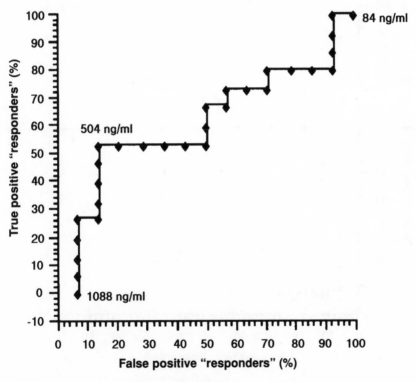

Figure 6–3. Receiver Operating Characteristic Curve (ROC) for the relationship between the Scale for the Assessment of Positive Symptoms (SAPS; Andreasen 1984) scores and clozapine plasma concentrations ranging from 84 to 1,088 ng/ml. True positive "responders," n = 15; false positive "responders," n = 14.

symptoms. Further, χ^2 analysis of these data revealed that differences between the responders and nonresponders at these particular minimal effective concentrations were significant ($\chi^2 = 4.887$, df = 1, $P = .027$). Likewise, a clozapine plasma concentration of 504 ng/ml or more demonstrated a sensitivity of 70% and a specificity of 74% for improvement in negative symptoms. The χ^2 analysis on the data found the differences between the responders and nonresponders at this particular minimal effective concentration significant ($\chi^2 = 5.154$, df = 1, $P = .02$). Finally, combining the SAPS and SANS global scores showed that again a plasma concentration of 504 ng/ml or more was the threshold level for an overall therapeutic response. Again χ^2 analysis found the differences between the responders and nonresponders significant ($\chi^2 = 7.635$, df = 1, $P = .006$). Similar to ob-

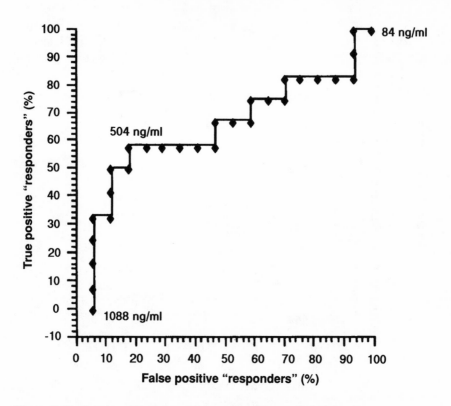

Figure 6–4. Receiver Operating Characteristic Curve (ROC) for the relationship between the Scale for the Assessment of Negative Symptoms (SANS; Andreasen 1983) scores and clozapine plasma concentrations ranging from 84 to 1,088 ng/ml. True positive "responders," $n = 12$; false positive "responders," $n = 17$.

servations using the BPRS analysis, the addition of the norclozapine concentration to the clozapine concentration did not change the outcome of any of the sensitivity and specificity findings. Table 6–2 demonstrates this observation. Thus laboratory measurement of norclozapine, one of the inactive metabolites of clozapine, is not necessary when monitoring clozapine therapy.

Perry et al. (1991a) found a 38% response rate to clozapine that was similar to the 30% rate found by Kane et al. (1988) in a 6-week, double-blind, multicenter trial. Meltzer et al. (1989) reported that 61% of treatment-resistant schizophrenic patients respond to clozapine when treated up to 12 months, suggesting that a trial of 6 weeks may not be adequate. Perry et al. (1991a) suggested that an alternative hypothesis to Meltzer's

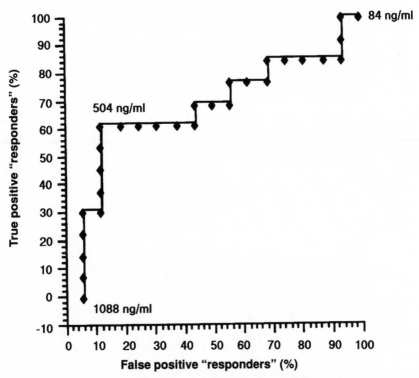

Figure 6–5. Receiver Operating Characteristic Curve (ROC) for the relationship between the Scale for the Assessment of Positive Symptoms (Andreason 1984) plus the Scale for the Assessment of Negative Symptoms (SANS; Andreasen 1983) scores and clozapine plasma concentrations ranging from 84 to 1,088 ng/ml. True positive "responders," $n = 13$; false positive "responders," $n = 16$.

Table 6–2. Receiver operating characteristic curve analyses to determine therapeutic clozapine concentrations

Rating scale	Drug	Threshold concentration (ng/ml)	Sensitivity (%)	Specificity (%)	χ^2	df	P
BPRS	Clozapine	397	64	78	4.974	1	.03
BPRS	Total clozapine	509	64	78	4.974	1	.03
SAPS	Clozapine	504	80	63	4.887	1	.03
SAPS	Total clozapine	609	80	63	4.887	1	.03
SANS	Clozapine	504	70	74	5.154	1	.02
SANS	Total clozapine	609	70	74	5.154	1	.02
SAPS + SANS	Clozapine	504	80	74	7.635	1	.006
SAPS + SANS	Total clozapine	609	80	74	7.635	1	.006

Note. BPRS = Brief Psychiatric Rating Scale (Overall and Gorham 1962); SAPS = Scale for the Assessment of Positive Symptoms (Andreasen 1984); SAPS = Scale for Assessment of Negative Symptoms (Andreasen 1983).

finding may be that initially the plasma concentrations were too low and when the dose was increased later the patients eventually responded. This explanation is reasonable when it is recalled that the response rate was 64% for patients with plasma clozapine concentrations greater than 397 ng/ml (Perry et al. 1991a).

Our analyses concluded that improvement in negative symptoms was most likely to occur in patients with clozapine plasma concentrations greater than 504 ng/ml. Perry et al. (1991a) previously reported that clozapine plasma concentrations greater than 350 ng/ml were associated with overall improvement as determined by the BPRS. In that analysis, the two positive symptom factors of the BPRS showed significantly greater decreases in the subjects who had clozapine concentrations of 350 ng/ml or more. The anergia factor on the BPRS appeared to improve regardless of the plasma concentrations. When the SAPS and SANS were used to assess the correlation between these plasma concentrations and therapeutic response, a clearer picture developed. With this more rigorous assessment of the primary symptoms of schizophrenia, it has been shown that improvement occurred most frequently in those patients with plasma concentrations of 504 ng/ml or more. As can be seen in Table 6–2, a clozapine plasma concentration of 504 ng/ml or more maximizes the predictive sensitivity and specificity of the clozapine plasma concentration measurement according to the combined assessments of the SAPS and SANS. The difference in sensitivity and specificity favoring the SAPS and SANS over the BPRS is not surprising. It is assumed that the difference is related to the ability of the SAPS and SANS to assess more specifically the individual positive and negative symptoms of schizophrenia, whereas the BPRS yields a more global measure.

By evaluating our SANS data, it was found that 41% (12 of 29) of the patients demonstrated improvement in their negative symptoms. Clozapine improved the negative symptoms of schizophrenia at a rate nearly as high as that for positive symptoms (52%). This is significant because typical neuroleptics exert their primary therapeutic effect on the positive symptoms of hallucinations and delusions and appear to have less effect on the negative symptoms. These data showed that the symptoms of alogia, anhedonia, and attention improved at a rate similar to the improvement rate for the positive symptoms. It was not possible to determine whether one group of symptoms improved first and caused the change in the other group, or if they were changing independently. This is particularly true because the SAPS and SANS are designed to reflect psychopathology that occurred during the past week. They do not measure changes that occur over shorter time periods. Since all the patients had significant positive symptoms at the start of the study, it is not surprising that those who demonstrated improvement had improvement in positive and negative symptoms. The decrease in positive and negative symptoms continued to be significant even when data from all subjects were included in the analysis. There was no correlation between the changes in affect and avolition and the change in positive symptoms, suggesting that these changes are independent.

On the basis of the present analysis of our data we concluded that a clozapine plasma concentration of 504 ng/ml or more is the optimum predictor of response to clozapine in treatment-refractory schizophrenic patients. Future research should be aimed at replicating these findings. Additionally, it would be useful to determine if smaller plasma concentrations of clozapine are effective in the treatment of schizophrenic patients who are not refractory to treatment.

References

Ackenheil M, Brau H, Burkhart A, et al: Antipsychoticsche wirksamkeit im verhaltnis zum plasmaspiegel von clozapine. Arzneimittelforsch (Drug Res) 26:1156–1158, 1976

Ackenheil M: Clozapine: pharmacokinetic investigations and biochemical effects in man. Psychopharmacology (Berl) 99:32–37, 1989

American Psychiatric Association: Diagnostic and Statistical Manual of Mental Disorders, 3rd Edition, Revised. Washington, DC, American Psychiatric Association, 1987

Andreasen NC: Negative symptoms in schizophrenia: definition and reliability. Arch Gen Psychiatry 39:784–788, 1982

Andreasen NC: The Scale for the Assessment of Negative Symptoms (SANS). Iowa City, IA, University of Iowa, 1983

Andreasen NC: The Scale for the Assessment of Positive Symptoms (SAPS). Iowa City, IA, University of Iowa, 1984

Brau H, Burkhart A, Pacha W, et al: Beziehungen zwischen wirkungen und plasmaspiegeln von clozapin. Arzneimittelforsch 28:1300, 1978

Guirguis E, Voineskos G, Gary J, et al: Clozapine (Leponex) versus chlorpromazine (Largactil) in acute schizophrenia (a double-blind study). Curr Ther Res 21:707–719, 1977

Guy W, Ban TA: The AMDP System: Manual for the Assessment and Documentation of Psychopathology. Heidelberg, Germany, Springer, 1982

Guy W, Cleray P, Bonato RR: Methodological implications of a large central data system. J Pharmacol 5 (suppl 1):13, 1974

Kane J, Honigfeld G, Singer J, et al: Clozapine for the treatment-resistant schizophrenic. A double-blind comparison with chlorpromazine. Arch Gen Psychiatry 45:489–496, 1988

Meltzer HY, Bastani B, Ramirez L, et al: Clozapine: new research on efficacy and mechanism of action. Eur Arch Psychiatr Neurol Sci 238:332–339, 1989

Mossman D, Somoza E: ROC curves, test accuracy, and the description of diagnostic tests. Journal of Neuropsychiatry and Clinical Neurosciences 3:330–333, 1991

Overall JE: The Brief Psychiatric Rating Scale in Psychopharmacology Research, in Pharmacopsychiatry, Vol 7. Edited by Pichot P. Basel, Switzerland, Karger, 1974

Perry PJ, Miller DD, Arndt SV, et al: Clozapine and norclozapine plasma concentrations and clinical response in treatment-refractory schizophrenics. Am J Psychiatry 148: 231–235, 1991a

Perry PJ, Miller DD, Arndt SV, et al. Clozapine concentrations and clinical response in schizophrenia (letter). Am J Psychiatry 148:1406–1407, 1991b

Shopsin B, Klein H, Aaronsom M, et al: Clozapine, chlorpromazine, and placebo in newly hospitalized, acutely schizophrenic patients. Arch Gen Psychiatry 36:657–664, 1979

Thorup M, Fog R: Clozapine treatment of schizophrenic patients. Plasma concentrations and coagulation factors. Acta Psychiatr Scand 55:123–126, 1977

CHAPTER 7

Plasma Level Monitoring for Long-Acting Injectable Neuroleptics

Stephen R. Marder, M.D.
Theodore Van Putten, M.D.
Manickam Aravagiri, Ph.D.
William C. Wirshing, M.D.
Kamal K. Midha, D.Sc.

L ong-acting injectable neuroleptics (LINs), or depot neuroleptics, are usually prescribed during the maintenance phase of treatment for schizophrenia. At this point, patients have either recovered from an acute psychotic episode or are in the process of recovering. The effectiveness of the depot drug is measured in terms of its ability to prevent psychotic relapse.

The monitoring of plasma levels of depot drugs during maintenance therapy could be particularly useful if it provided an objective method of assessing a patient's pharmacotherapy. Decisions about drug dose during this phase are particularly problematic because the clinician is unable to assess a clinical response in individuals who are clinically stable. The clinician will usually select a drug dose and wait to see if the patient relapses as the result of too little drug or develops side effects as the result of too high a dose. There is often a lengthy interval between the time the decision is made and when it can be interpreted. For example, studies suggest that

Supported by the Department of Veterans Affairs Medical Research Service and the UCLA Mental Health Clinical Research Center for the Study of Schizophrenia (National Institute of Mental Health).

when a placebo is substituted for an active neuroleptic, the majority of relapses will occur from 4 to 7 months later. Under these circumstances, a plasma level could provide reassurance that a patient is receiving an adequate amount of drug.

Plasma level measurements could also provide guidance to clinicians who are trying to treat patients with the lowest effective neuroleptic dose. Recent studies (Kane et al. 1983; Marder et al. 1987; Hogarty et al. 1988) have suggested that a proportion of chronic schizophrenic patients can be treated with doses of neuroleptics substantially lower than those usually prescribed. However, lowering the dose in a stabilized individual may increase that person's risk of relapsing. Dose reduction strategies might be carried out more safely if plasma level measurements could provide the treating physician with an indication that the patients may be receiving an inadequate dose.

Problems in Studying Plasma Levels in Maintenance Therapy

LINs, or depot neuroleptics, have certain characteristics that make them considerably more difficult to study than oral drugs. One of those characteristics is the length of time it takes these drugs to reach a steady-state level. Figure 7–1 is from a study in our laboratory in which chronic schizophrenic patients were randomly assigned to either 5 or 25 mg of fluphenazine decanoate administered every 2 weeks (Marder et al. 1987). Fluphenazine levels were measured at regular intervals using a radioimmunoassay (RIA) developed by Midha and his colleagues at the University of Saskatchewan (McKay et al. 1983; Midha et al. 1980). The most important data comes from the group of patients randomly assigned to the higher dose. On the 25-mg dose, patients required as long as 3 to 6 months to reach a steady-state level. Others (McCreadie et al. 1986; Gelders 1986) have reported similar results for haloperidol decanoate, although Deberdt et al. (1980) reported that haloperidol reached a steady-state level in patients after only two monthly injections.

The length of time that it takes LINs to reach a steady-state level can be a significant problem for researchers and clinicians. The researcher should be cautious about interpreting a plasma level during the first several weeks of treatment because the patient may not be at steady-state level. At this stage, plasma levels may be rising if the patient had a dose increase in the past several months or falling if, for example, the patient has recently been changed from a higher dose of an oral to a depot drug. As a result, it may be incorrect to associate the plasma level with the depot dose or the immediate clinical course with a changing plasma concentration. It is important, therefore, that clinicians design studies that provide assurance that patients are at steady-state level when plasma concentrations are measured. This is not a completely satisfactory resolution for a number of reasons. First, it requires that patients be followed for long study intervals. In our previously mentioned study (Marder et al. 1991) we waited 3 months and then measured plasma level–clinical outcome relationships during the next year and 9 months. Another important disadvantage is that patients who relapse before they reach steady-state levels are eliminated from the analysis.

Another problem in maintenance studies is the assay sensitivity that may be required. Patients are usually treated with substantially lower drug doses during maintenance therapy. This creates an obvious problem for measuring some neuroleptic plasma concentrations. The most obvious example is fluphenazine. A number of studies indicate that acutely ill patients

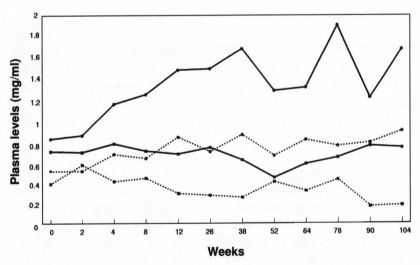

Figure 7–1. Mean fluphenazine (*solid line*) and fluphenazine sulfoxide (*dotted line*) levels for patients who remained on their original fixed dose of 5 mg or 25 mg of fluphenazine decanoate at each time point.
Source. Reprinted from Marder SR, Midha KK, Van Putten T, et al: "Plasma Levels of Fluphenazine in Patients Receiving Fluphenazine Decanoate: Relationship to Clinical Response." *British Journal of Psychiatry* 158:658–665, 1991. Used with permission of *British Journal of Psychiatry*.

commonly have a clinical response but have plasma levels in the subnanogram range (Dudley et al. 1983; Dysken et al. 1981; Mavroidis et al. 1984; Tune et al. 1980). Plasma levels may be considerably lower for patients treated with fluphenazine decanoate. For this reason, studies of fluphenazine plasma levels have often required the sensitivity of a RIA.

It is important to add that data about effective plasma levels for oral neuroleptics should not be generalized to studies of depot drugs. This is because there are significant differences in the kinetics of oral and depot drugs. When a drug is taken orally it is less bioavailable than when it is administered parenterally as a depot injection. This is partly because of variability in drug absorption but more importantly because of the extensive metabolism that orally administered neuroleptics, particularly phenothiazines such as fluphenazine, undergo during the first pass through the gut and liver. Differences among patients in these factors can result in large differences in the amount of oral drug that patients may require to maintain a particular plasma level. In addition, some of the activity of an administered neuroleptic may be because of active metabolites that are not measured by most chemical assay methods. As a result, studies of the clinical effects associated with plasma concentrations should be carried out separately for oral and depot neuroleptics (Marder et al. 1989).

Among the problems in maintenance-therapy studies is the measurement of outcome. In studies of patients with acute psychosis, clinicians can compare the amount of improvement or the lack of it that occurs at different plasma levels. In maintenance-therapy studies, patients begin the study in a stable condition and the clinician is forced to measure a negative outcome, which is psychotic relapse or exacerbation. In contrast to acute studies, there are no widely accepted standards for measuring relapse rate. Early studies of maintenance therapy used hospitalization or the imminent need for hospitalization as the definition of relapse. However, the need for hospitalization is often determined by factors that are unrelated to the patient's schizophrenic symptoms. Moreover, if the investigator waits until a severe event such as a relapse occurs, individuals may suffer serious losses such as damage to their personal relationships or loss of self-esteem. As a result, more recent studies (Marder et al. 1987; Hogarty et al. 1988) have used milder manifestations of a recurrence of psychosis. Our study (Marder et al. 1987) defined negative outcome as a psychotic exacerbation that was defined in terms of a worsening on psychosis items from the Brief Psychiatric Rating Scale (BPRS).

The measurement of side effects and compliance take on great importance in maintenance studies. A degree of extrapyramidal and other side effects may be tolerable for patients who are being treated for a severe psychotic state. In contrast, even mild effects may be unacceptable for individuals who are living in the community and who experience them for weeks and months. Moreover, there is evidence that extrapyramidal effects, particularly akathisia and akinesia, can be difficult to differentiate from other symptoms (Van Putten and Marder 1987). For example, mild akathisia can be difficult to distinguish from anxiety, and akinesia can mimic negative symptoms of schizophrenia. Because one of the important goals of maintenance therapy is to facilitate patient rehabilitation, the occurrence of even mild side effects should be considered an important outcome to be measured in relation to depot neuroleptic plasma levels.

One of the more serious manifestations of side effects can be noncompliance. Although prescribing depot drugs can substantially improve compliance in outpatient populations, excessive doses and perhaps excessive plasma concentrations can lead patients to leave treatment. As a result, drop-out rates are also important outcome measures to relate to plasma concentrations.

Studies of Fluphenazine Plasma Levels and Clinical Response

Relatively few studies have focused on the value of measuring fluphenazine levels in patients treated with fluphenazine decanoate. Wistedt et al. (1982) studied levels of fluphenazine and a metabolite, 7-hydroxyfluphenazine, in patients who received fluphenazine decanoate (mean dose, 21.4 mg every 2 weeks). Patients who relapsed had lower plasma levels (mean, 0.92 ng/ml) than those who did not relapse (mean, 1.36 ng/ml).

We recently studied fluphenazine plasma levels in patients who were randomly assigned to either 5 or 25 mg of fluphenazine decanoate every 2 weeks in a double-blind comparison (Marder et al. 1991). Patients were men who fulfilled DSM-III criteria (American Psychiatric Association 1980) for schizophrenia and who could be stabilized on 25 mg or less of fluphenazine decanoate every 2 weeks. After a stable period, subjects were placed on their assigned dose and monitored for 2 years with measures of clinical psychopathology and side effects. When patients demonstrated a worsening on BPRS cluster scores of three or more for thought disturbance or paranoia they were considered to have had a psychotic exacerbation. Most exacerbations were rather mild and easily managed by an increase in the patient's fluphenazine decanoate dose.

Blood samples for plasma level measurements were drawn at 2, 3, 6, 9, 12, 15, 18, and 24 months following randomly assigning patients to treatment groups. Samples were drawn 2 weeks after the previous injection and just before the next injection was administered. Plasma levels of fluphenazine were measured using RIA (Midha et al. 1980) that was validated for specificity using gas chromatography-mass spectroscopy (Dudley et al. 1983). The sensitivity of the fluphenazine method was 0.1 ng/ml and the coefficient of variation was 3%. The antisera used for the RIA did not cross-react with benztropine or other commonly used antiparkinsonian drugs.

We compared relapse risk with plasma concentrations that were reached after patients achieved steady-state levels. For all analyses, plasma concentrations were log transformed. Therefore, levels at 3, 6, and 9 months following randomly assigning patients to treatment groups were measured and we studied the relationship of plasma fluphenazine concentration and the rate of psychotic exacerbations during the subsequent year.

Using logistic regression, the relationship between plasma concentration and exacerbation risk was nonsignificant at 3 months ($\chi^2 = .21$, df = 1, $P = .65$) but significant at 6 months ($\chi^2 = 4.38$, df = 1, $P = .04$) and 9 months ($\chi^2 = 6.62$, df = 1, $P = .003$) (Figures 7–2 and 7–3). (The sample size was too small at later time points for meaningful analysis.) The same relationship was apparent when the mean plasma levels were compared for patients who exacerbated and those who did not. At 6 months, the mean fluphenazine plasma level for patients who did exacerbate was 0.62 (standard deviation [SD], .47) and for patients who did not exacerbate it was 1.33 (SD, 1.04, $P = .01$). At 9 months, the mean fluphenazine plasma level for patients who did exacerbate was 0.51 (SD, .36) and for patients who did not exacerbate it was 1.59 (SD, 1.27, $P = .001$) (Figure 7–4).

The relationship between plasma levels and the rate of psychotic exacerbations over the subsequent 12-month period was also studied by survival analysis using the log-transformed fluphenazine levels as a covariate (Cox models). This is a more sensitive method of data analysis compared with logistic regression because it takes into account the length of time between the index evaluation (at 3, 6, and 9 months) and the week in which the patient exacerbates. Using this method, we found a relationship between the fluphenazine plasma level and the risk of exacerbations at 6 months that was nearly statistically significant ($\chi^2 = 3.77$, df = 1, $P = .052$) and a relationship at 9 months that was significant ($\chi^2 = 11.25$, df = 1, $P = .0008$). At 3 months, the relationship was nonsignificant ($\chi^2 = .87$, df = 1, $P = .65$).

We also studied the relationship between plasma concentrations of fluphenazine and neurological side effects. Although we found significant correlations at some points (2, 4, and 26 weeks) between akinesia and fluphenazine levels, this relationship was inconsistent and was not present with other side effects. This lack of a relationship may be explained by a previously reported finding that patients who experienced the most side effects tended to be the patients who dropped out of the study (Marder et al. 1987).

It is interesting to note that these results are somewhat inconsistent with the results from studies with oral fluphenazine. For example, Mavroidis et al. (1984) found that patients receiving oral fluphenazine for the treatment of acute psychotic episodes responded well in the dose range of 0.13–0.70 ng/ml. Dysken et al. (1981) reported that fluphenazine levels above 0.2 ng/ml appeared to be effective. The lower levels found effective in these studies do not necessarily contradict our findings because the low

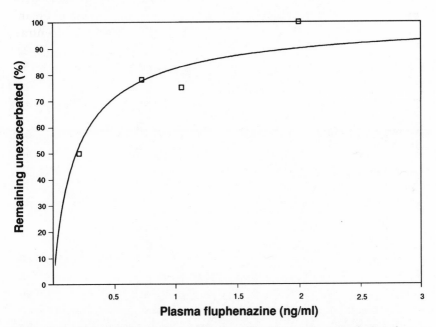

Figure 7–2. Relationship between risk of psychotic exacerbations during the following year and plasma fluphenazine levels at 6 months ($n = 33$). The line represents the logistic regression function computed from the actual data ($\chi^2 = 4.38$, df = 1, $P = .04$). The squares represent the actual percent remaining stable in each quartile, displayed at the quartile midpoint.

Source. Reprinted from Marder SR, Midha KK, Van Putten T, et al: "Plasma Levels of Fluphenazine in Patients Receiving Fluphenazine Decanoate: Relationship to Clinical Response." *British Journal of Psychiatry* 158:658–665, 1991. Used with permission of *British Journal of Psychiatry.*

levels of fluphenazine they found may result from the extensive metabolism of oral fluphenazine. Conceivably, these patients may have had higher levels of fluphenazine metabolites such as 7-hydroxyfluphenazine or fluphenazine-N-oxide that may have accounted for the effectiveness of the oral dose.

Although these results clearly need to be replicated, they strongly suggest that measuring plasma levels of fluphenazine may be useful for patients in long-term maintenance treatment. As shown in Figures 7–2 and 7–3, rates of psychotic exacerbation were relatively low when fluphenazine plasma levels were above 0.8 or 0.9 ng/ml, which suggests that this is a reasonable level for maintenance. However, very few patients with plasma levels above 1.2 ng/ml exhibited exacerbations, which suggests that if the clinician had given a priority to preventing relapse and was less concerned

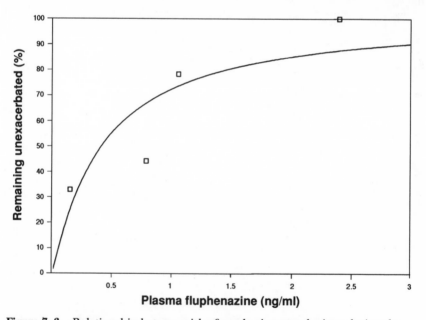

Figure 7–3. Relationship between risk of psychotic exacerbations during the following year and plasma fluphenazine levels at 9 months ($n = 35$). The line represents the logistic regression function computed from the actual data ($\chi^2 = 8.98$, df = 1; $P = .003$). The squares represent the actual percent remaining stable in each quartile, displayed at the quartile midpoint.
Source. Reprinted from Marder SR, Midha KK, Van Putten T, et al: "Plasma Levels of Fluphenazine in Patients Receiving Fluphenazine Decanoate: Relationship to Clinical Response." *British Journal of Psychiatry* 158:658–665, 1991. Used with permission of *British Journal of Psychiatry.*

about side effects, then the higher level might be preferable. In contrast, patients with fluphenazine plasma levels that are lower than 0.9 ng/ml may be on the linear part of the curve and would benefit from a dose increase. Patients who received 25 mg of fluphenazine decanoate every 2 weeks had mean levels of about 1.4 ng/ml and nearly all were statistically on the flatter part of the curve. Patients receiving a 5-mg dose in our study (Marder 1991) had mean fluphenazine plasma levels of 0.6 to 0.7 ng/ml with standard deviations of 0.5 to 0.6, indicating that this dose led to a substantial number of patients having levels that rendered them vulnerable to psychotic exacerbations.

There are a number of circumstances in which plasma level measurements of fluphenazine could have potential use. If patients experience side effects on a particular dose of fluphenazine decanoate, plasma level measurements could be used to titrate the patient's dose down to a lower dose that would provide adequate protection. Similarly, if a clinician was lower-

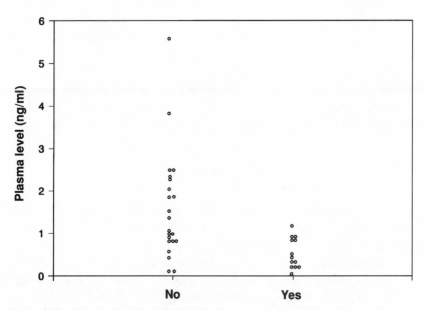

Figure 7–4. Plasma fluphenazine levels drawn at 9 months in patients who experienced exacerbations (mean level, 0.51 ng/ml; SD, .36) and those who did not (mean level, 1.59 ng/ml; SD 1.27; t test, P = .001). *Source.* Reprinted from Marder SR, Midha KK, Van Putten T, et al: "Plasma Levels of Fluphenazine in Patients Receiving Fluphenazine Decanoate: Relationship to Clinical Response." *British Journal of Psychiatry* 158:658–665, 1991. Used with permission of *British Journal of Psychiatry.*

ing the dose of a neuroleptic in order to reduce the risk of tardive dyskinesia or to reduce the amount of akinesia, plasma level monitoring would provide some assurance that the patient was receiving an adequate amount of drug to prevent exacerbation. One of the possible benefits of using plasma level measurements would be to give clinicians confidence that they could safely lower fluphenazine decanoate doses.

Plasma Levels of Other Depot Neuroleptics

There are relatively few studies of plasma levels with other depot neuroleptics. For example, there are no controlled, fixed-dose studies comparing levels of haloperidol and clinical response in patients receiving haloperidol decanoate. In contrast, there is substantial literature indicating a relationship between plasma levels of haloperidol and clinical response in patients who receive oral haloperidol. There may be problems in generalizing from studies of oral neuroleptics to depot drugs because of the differences in drug metabolism between the two routes of administration. However, the oral bioavailability of haloperidol is much greater than that of fluphenazine, and reduced haloperidol has substantially less activity than the parent drug. As a result, measuring the parent compound probably provides similar information for depot and oral formulations. If this is the case, then haloperidol plasma levels of 5–15 ng/ml may define the therapeutic range.

Conclusions

Studies relating clinical response to plasma levels have usually focused on the acute stage of treatment and have used oral neuroleptics. However, it may turn out that the most routine application of plasma level measurement will be for long-term treatment. The reasons are twofold: first, during maintenance therapy the physician is unable to titrate clinical response against drug dose because patients are usually clinically stable and the results of too low a dose may not be apparent for months. Second, clinicians are usually interested in treating patients with the lowest effective dose as a means of minimizing both acute extrapyramidal symptoms and the risk of tardive dyskinesia. Plasma level measurements may provide objective information that encourages clinicians to lower doses. At the same time, long-acting depot drugs are probably the preferred route of administration for most patients who are receiving maintenance neuroleptics. In addition, during the next several years a number of atypical neuroleptics, such as clozapine, will become available in the United States. None of these is likely to be available as a depot compound. Therefore, clinicians will be motivated to prescribe long-acting drugs as safely and effectively as possible.

References

American Psychiatric Association: Diagnostic and Statistical Manual of Mental Disorders, 3rd Edition. Washington, DC American Psychiatric Association, 1980

Deberdt R, Elens W, Berghmans J, et al: Intramuscular haloperidol decanoate for neuroleptic maintenance therapy: efficacy, dosage schedule, and plasma levels. Acta Psychiatr Scand 62:356–363, 1980

Dudley J, Rauw G, Hawes EM, et al: Correlation of fluphenazine plasma levels versus clinical response in patients: a pilot study. Prog Neuropsychopharmacol Biol Psychiatry 207:791–795, 1983

Dysken MW, Javaid JI, Chang SS, et al: Fluphenazine pharmacokinetics and therapeutic response. Psychopharmacology (Berl) 73:205–210, 1981

Gelders YG: Pharmacology, pharmacokinetics and clinical development of haloperidol decanoate. Int Clin Psychopharmacol 1(s):1–11, 1986

Hogarty GE, McEvoy JP, Munetz M, et al: Dose of fluphenazine, familial expressed emotion, and outcome in schizophrenia: results of a two-year controlled study. Arch Gen Psychiatry 45:797–805, 1988

Kane JM, Rifkin A, Woerner M, et al: Low dose neuroleptic treatment of outpatient schizophrenics: I. Preliminary results for relapse rates. Arch Gen Psychiatry 40:893–896, 1983

Marder SR, Van Putten T, Mintz J, et al: Low and conventional dose maintenance therapy with fluphenazine decanoate: two year outcome. Arch Gen Psychiatry 44:518–521, 1987

Marder SR, Hubbard JW, Van Putten T, et al: The pharmacokinetics of long-acting injectable neuroleptic drugs: Clinical implications. Psychopharmacology (Berl) 98:433–439, 1989

Marder SR, Midha KK, Van Putten T, et al: Plasma levels of fluphenazine in patients receiving fluphenazine decanoate: relationship to clinical response. Brit J Psychiatry 158:658–665, 1991

Mavroidis ML, Kanter DR, Hirschowitz J, et al: Fluphenazine plasma levels and clinical response. J Clin Psychiatry 45:370–373, 1984

McCreadie RG, McKane JP, Robinson ADT, et al: Depot neuroleptics as maintenance therapy in chronic schizophrenic in-patients. Int Clin Psychopharmacol 1(s):13–14, 1986

McKay G, Hall K, Eden R, et al: Subnanogram determination of fluphenazine in human plasma by gas chromatography mass spectrometry. Biomed Mass Spectrom 10:550–555, 1983

Midha KK, Cooper JK, Hubbard JW: Radioimmunoassay for fluphenazine in human plasma. Commun Psychopharmacol 4:107–114, 1980

Tune LE, Creese I, Depaulo JR, et al: Clinical state and serum neuroleptic levels measured by radioreceptor assay in schizophrenia. Am J Psychiatry 137:187–190, 1980

Van Putten T, Marder SR: Behavioral toxicity of antipsychotic drugs. J Clin Psychiatry 48 (suppl):13–19, 1987

Wistedt B, Jorgensen A, Wiles D: A depot neuroleptic withdrawal study: plasma concentration of fluphenazine and flupenthixol and relapse frequency. Psychopharmacology (Berl) 78:301–304, 1982

CHAPTER 8

Neuroleptic Plasma Concentrations

An Estimate of Their Sensitivity and Specificity as a Predictor of Response

Paul J. Perry, Ph.D.
Daniel A. Smith, Pharm.D.

The clinical value of employing antipsychotic plasma concentrations as a monitor for drug doses for schizophrenic patients is a widely debated and complicated issue. Numerous reviews with varying opinions have been written over the years. Routine plasma level monitoring of neuroleptics has clinical utility for several reasons. Interindividual pharmacokinetic variation usually makes it unrealistic to adjust patient dose based on a by-weight basis. Excessively high concentrations of a drug may be associated with clinical deterioration of the patient because of increased adverse effects and neuroleptic toxicity. Additionally, plasma level monitoring assures compliance. The intent of this chapter is to identify, review, and summarize the neuroleptic blood level clinical studies with technically appropriate design and methodology. Additionally, an internal analysis was conducted for those studies that supplied sufficient raw data. To determine if a relationship existed between the plasma concentration of the neuroleptic and therapeutic response, Receiver Operating Characteristic (ROC) curves were generated and the sensitivity and specificity of the blood level data was assessed using χ^2 analyses. The utility of this analytical methodology has been demonstrated in evaluating haloperidol (Kelly et al. 1990) and clozapine data (Perry et al. 1991).

For a study to be considered for review and further analysis several minimum criteria had to be met. First, to establish a reasonably homogeneous diagnostic set of patients, a diagnosis indicating schizophrenia was required. It has been our experience in analyzing neuroleptic blood level data with mixed diagnostic patient populations (e.g., schizophrenic, schizophreniform, and schizoaffective) that the results of an analysis can change considerably when only schizophrenic patients are considered alone without inclusion of all psychotic patients. Thus, the preferred diagnostic criteria for schizophrenia included Research Diagnostic Criteria (RDC; Spitzer et al. 1978), DSM-III (American Psychiatric Association 1980), or DSM-III-R (American Psychiatric Association 1987). Exceptions to this rule were made for some of the older studies that were performed before the use of these criteria was widespread. Furthermore, only studies in which acutely ill patients were treated were considered. Next, the study was required to utilize a fixed dose of neuroleptic for a minimum of 2 weeks. Studies that allow upward dose titration during the observation period always bias the results toward a curvilinear relationship. A validated psychosis rating scale such as the Brief Psychiatric Rating Scale (BPRS; Overall and Gorham 1962) or the New Haven Schizophrenic Index (NHSI; Astrachan et al. 1972) was essential to quantify psychopathology.

Acceptable neuroleptic assay methodology included highly specific assays such as high-performance liquid chromatography (HPLC), gas-liquid (GLC) chromatography, and radioimmunoassays (RIA). The radioreceptor assay (RRA) was not acceptable. The RRA measures the total dopamine receptor-blocking activity in the blood and therefore accounts for not only parent drug but active metabolites as well. Neuroleptic blood-to-brain distribution ratios may differ between neuroleptics because of differences in protein binding in the plasma and the cerebrospinal fluid (CSF). Because only free and unbound drug are active in the brain, the plasma RRA may not adequately mirror the amount of active free drug in the central nervous system. It was not surprising that a review of these studies concluded that RRA assays were not a useful tool for plasma concentration monitoring of neuroleptics (Dahl 1986). Thus, studies using RRA were excluded from this review.

For our internal analysis, the optimal split or cutoff point for the neuroleptic concentrations was estimated by drawing ROC curves (Mossman and Somoza 1991). ROC curves are ideal for this purpose because they provide an objective method to identify the threshold neuroleptic plasma concentration needed for response. To construct a ROC curve, the percentage of "true positive responders" (i.e., the proportion of responsive patients at a particular drug concentration) is plotted on the y-axis against the percentage of "false positive responders" (i.e., the proportion of non-responsive patients at a particular drug concentration) on the x-axis. The ROC curve designates an optimum cutoff point that is characterized by the parameters of sensitivity (true positive rate) and specificity (true negative rate).

Unlike the original analyses (Kelly et al. 1990; Perry et al. 1991), the ROC curves constructed to analyze the data considered in this review graphed each data point separately. The original data graphed haloperidol and clozapine plasma concentration ranges rather than each point separately. The figurative representation of the data in this chapter present a more precise illustration of the maximum sensitivity/specificity point. ROC curves usually do not graph each point separately but utilize ranges as was done in the original studies. The optimum predictive plasma concentration on a ROC curve is located at the point closest to the true positive responder y-axis and furthest from the false positive responder x-axis. Oftentimes this point is less than obvious when the data are visually inspected. Thus the optimum sensitivity point on the graph is that point that has the largest difference when the false positive responder value (x) is subtracted from true positive responder value (y). This point identifies the drug concentration that maximizes sensitivity and specificity for the drug concentration response marker. The identification of an optimum cutoff point results in the data being practically divided into four categories or rates: true positives, false positives, true negatives, and false negatives. These four rates are the same as those yielded by the 2×2 matrix of a contingency table constructed for a χ^2 analysis. The sensitivity (true positive rate, i.e., ++ cell) and specificity (true negative rate, i.e., – – cell) for the cutoff point are then determined by performing a χ^2 analysis to determine if the distribution is significantly different between the four cells.

A 30% reduction in psychopathology was used as an *a priori* criterion of response unless another measure was specified by the authors of the studies reviewed. Table 8–1 presents the characteristics for the studies utilized in the ROC analyses. Table 8–2 presents the recommended therapeutic ranges for each study along with the sensitivity and specificity values for those data.

Chlorpromazine

Historically, chlorpromazine is the prototypical neuroleptic used for the treatment of schizophrenia. The search for a relationship between chlor-

Table 8–1. Characteristics of therapeutic-response studies

Study	Drug	Diagnostic criteria	n	Age range (years)	Sex (M:F)	Drug-free (weeks)	Rating scale	Dose (mg/day)	Duration (weeks)	Assay Type	CV (%)	Sensitivity (ng/ml)
Magliozzi et al. (1981)	Hal	RDC	10	16–54	6:4	2	BPRS	2–30	3–12	GLC	5	1
Garver et al. (1984)	Hal	DSM-III	14	NA	NA	>3 days	NHSI	6;12;24	2	GLC	1.2–5.9	0.2
Linkowski et al. (1984)	Hal	DSM-III	20	19–53	11:9	>1	BPRS	30	6	RIA	3	NA
Santos et al. (1989)	Hal	DSM-III	30	26 ± 6	NA	≥10	BPRS	10;15;30	3	RIA	13.7	0.05
Kelly et al. (1990)	Hal	DSM-III	29	17–56	19:10	Several days to weeks	BPRS	8–18 ng/ml or 25 ng/ml	2	HPLC	5–8	2
Bigelow et al. (1985)	Hal	DSM-III	19	20–41	14:5	6	BPRS psychosis factor	0.4 mg/kg body weight per day	6	HPLC	NA	NA

Study												
Van Putten et al. (1985)	Hal	NA	33	NA	NA	Several days to weeks	BPRS psychosis factor	5;10; or 20	4	RIA	NA	NA
Janicak et al. (1989)	Tri	RDC	30	19–78	NA	3–36 days	BPRS	10	2	GLC	6.7	0.2
Mavroidis et al. (1984a)	Thi	DSM-III	19	NA	NA	NA	NHSI	16; 30; or 60	2	GLC	NA	NA
Mavroidis et al. (1984b)	Flu	DSM-III	19	NA	NA	NA	NHSI	5;10; or 20	2	GLC	NA	NA
Levinson et al. (1988)	Flu	RDC	22	NA	NA	NA	BPRS thought disturbance	10 or 20	24 days	RIA	NA	NA
Perry et al. (1991)	Clo	DSM-III-R	29	19–48	20:9	Most >3 weeks	BPRS	250;300;350; 400; or 450	4	HPLC	0.9–4.2	50

Note. CV = Coefficient of variation; Hal = haloperidol; Tri = trifluoperazine; Thi = thiothixene; Flu = fluphenazine; Clo = clozapine; NA = not available; BW = body weight; RDC = Research Diagnostic Criteria (Spitzer et al. 1978); DSM-III (American Psychiatric Association 1980); DSM-III-R (American Psychiatric Association 1987); BPRS = Brief Psychiatric Rating Scale (Overall and Gorham 1962); NHSI = New Haven Schizophenic Index (Astrachan et al. 1972); GLC = gas-liquid chromatography; RIA = radioimmunoassay; HPLC = high-performance liquid chromatography.

Table 8–2. Receiver operating characteristic (ROC) curve analyses to determine therapeutic range

Study	Drug	Lower limit					Upper limit				
		(ng/ml)	Sensitivity	Specificity	χ^2	P	(ng/ml)	Sensitivity	Specificity	χ^2	P
Linkowski et al. (1984)	Hal	9.5	87%	60%	4.36	.04	None	NA	NA	NA	NA
Magliozzi et al. (1981)	Hal	8	80%	100%	6.67	.01	None	NA	NA	NA	NA
Garver et al. (1984)	Hal	5	100%	75%	7.87	.005	14	100%	75%	7.87	.005
Santos et al. (1989)	Hal	9	86%	63%	12.14	<.0005	None	NA	NA	NA	NA
Kelly et al. (1990)	Hal	None	NA	NA	NA	NA	15	55%	83%	4.58	.03
Bigelow et al. (1985)	Hal	18	83%	31%	.42	.52	None	NA	NA	NA	NA
Van Putten et al. (1985)	Hal	2.0	52%	100%	6.17	.013	None	NA	NA	NA	NA
Janicak et al. (1989)	Tri	1.05	70%	100%	18.26	<.0001	2.25	70%	100%	18.26	<.0001
Mavroidis et al. (1984a)	Thi	1.7	100%	69%	7.89	.005	10.5	100%	69%	7.89	.005
Mavroidis et al. (1984b)	Flu	2.3	75%	46%	.61	.45	None	NA	NA	NA	NA
Perry et al. (1991)	Clo	397	64%	78%	4.97	.03	None	NA	NA	NA	NA

Note. Hal = haloperidol; Tri = trifluoperazine; Thi = thiothixene; Flu = fluphenazine; Clo = clozapine; NA = not applicable.

promazine serum concentrations and response in schizophrenia is complicated by a lack of well-designed studies. Only two studies met our inclusion criteria for consideration in this review (Wode-Helgodt et al. 1978; Van Putten et al. 1981). Unfortunately, internal analysis of these data was not possible because the raw data were not reported in either of these studies.

Wode-Helgodt et al. (1978) performed the first fixed-dose study to identify a relationship between chlorpromazine blood concentrations and response in 48 acutely psychotic schizophrenic patients. Following baseline measurements during a week-long placebo phase, the patients were assigned to a fixed dose of either 200, 400, or 600 mg/day for 4 weeks of treatment. Psychopathology was assessed at baseline, 2 weeks, and 4 weeks using the sum of six items on the Comprehensive Psychopathological Rating Scale (CPRS; Asberg et al. 1978). In evaluations of 31 patients a significant inverse relationship was found between chlorpromazine blood and CSF concentrations and CPRS score at week 2 but not at week 4. Significant threshold CSF and plasma concentrations of 1 ng/ml and 40 ng/ml were identified as cut points above which a positive response was more likely when a 50% decrease in CPRS score was used as a measure of response. Unfortunately, it is impossible to identify those patients who experienced a 50% reduction in symptoms from the data presented. Interpretation of this data is difficult because only six patients had a chlorpromazine concentration above 1 ng/ml and 40 ng/ml in the CSF and plasma, respectively. The remaining 25 patients had chlorpromazine concentrations below these values. Clearly, there were many responders at concentrations below these cut points, indicating that the specificity of these threshold values is not very high. As a result, these threshold values are not very useful clinically because many patients may respond at chlorpromazine plasma concentrations below 40 ng/ml.

Van Putten et al. (1981) studied 47 acutely ill schizophrenic patients and 1 schizoaffective patient with a fixed dose of 6.6 mg/kg body weight per day of chlorpromazine for 28 days. Although one of the patients was diagnosed with schizoaffective disorder, this study was included in this review because of the small number of adequate chlorpromazine blood concentration studies. Response was defined as a decrease of 6 points or more in the BPRS score at the end of the 28-day fixed-dose period. The utility of this measure of response is questionable because a 6-point decrease of a typical baseline BPRS of 45 would only be a 13% decrease in symptomatology. Of the 34 patients who finished the 28-day fixed-dose phase, 18 were classified as "responders" and 16 as "nonresponders." Chlorpromazine plasma concentrations ranged from 3–207 ng/ml in the responsive patients and 0–227 ng/ml in the nonresponsive patients. However, the three responsive patients with the highest chlorpromazine concentrations (ranging from 105–207 ng/ml) experienced many side effects including hypotension, sedation, blurred vision, and phototoxicity. Eleven of the nonresponsive patients were treated openly for another 28 days at higher chlorpromazine doses. Four of five of these patients responded with blood concentrations less than 72 ng/ml. None of the six remaining patients with chlorpromazine plasma concentrations above 95 ng/ml responded. These results led the authors to propose an upper limit for therapeutic effect in most patients as 72 ng/ml. A lower limit for therapeutic effect could not be determined. These findings cast further doubt on the study of Wode-Helgodt et al. (1978) because 11 of the responsive patients and 11 of the nonresponsive patients had chlorpromazine concentrations below 40 ng/ml.

The results from these two studies indicate that a therapeutic range for chlorpromazine is far from established. The role of active metabolites also needs to be elucidated. Furthermore, it is unlikely that appropriately designed studies of chlorpromazine blood concentrations will be conducted because interest in neuroleptics has shifted to newer agents. It is recommended that clinicians continue to administer chlorpromazine in an empirical fashion.

Haloperidol

By far, haloperidol is the most extensively studied neuroleptic in the research describing a relationship between blood levels and therapeutic response. There are seven studies available that contain sufficient data and met the criteria to allow analysis using ROCs.

Magliozzi et al. (1981) examined the relationship between haloperidol concentration and response in 11 patients with diagnoses of schizophrenia according to RDC. One patient was excluded for failing to meet fixed-dose criteria. The remaining 10 patients were treated with fixed doses of 2 to 30 mg/day for 3 to 12 weeks. Patients received no haloperidol for 2 weeks before the start of the trial. Response was measured as a function of the total BPRS score. This was the only study that utilized the European version of the BPRS (0–6 scoring scale) rather than the American version (1–7 scoring scale). The scores were converted to the American BPRS scaling system to preserve the homogeneity of the internal analysis. Five (50%) responsive patients could be identified using a 30% decline in total BPRS scores as a measure of response. Blood levels ranged from 0–16.0 ng/ml. Our ROC curve identifies a concentration of 8 ng/ml as threshold of response (Figure 8–1). This finding was significant by χ^2 analysis ($\chi^2 = 6.67$, df = 1, $P = 0.01$). The sensitivity and specificity for haloperidol concentrations of 8 ng/ml or more as a clinical predictor of response were 80% and 100%, respectively. There was no obvious upper limit defining therapeutic response.

Garver et al. (1984) administered haloperidol doses of 6, 12, or 24 mg/d for 2 weeks to 14 schizophrenic patients experiencing an acute exacerbation of symptoms. Changes in psychotic symptoms were assessed using the NHSI. A 30% decline in the NHSI was observed in 8 (57%) of the patients. Haloperidol plasma levels ranged from 1–21 ng/ml. The authors

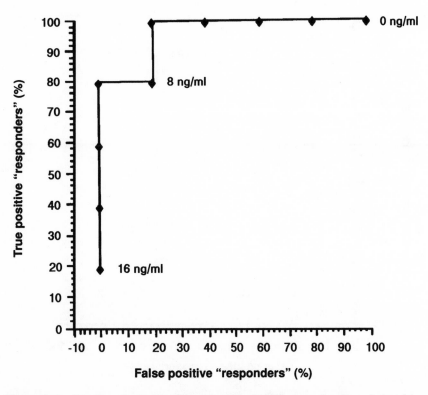

Figure 8–1. Receiver Operating Characteristic (ROC) curve for the relationship between Brief Psychiatric Rating Scale (BPRS; Overall and Gorham 1962) scores and haloperidol plasma concentrations ranging from 0 to 16 ng/ml for the Magliozzi et al. (1981) data set. True positive "responders," $n = 5$; false positive "responders," $n = 5$.

reported a significant curvilinear relationship with the therapeutic plasma levels proposed to range between 3–11 ng/ml. As can be seen in Figure 8–2, the shape of this ROC curve is sigmoidal rather than the usual exponential shape. This indicates that the data set is linear rather than curvilinear. Similar to Figure 8–1, Figure 8–2 defines the lower limit for a therapeutic response at 4 ng/ml. In order to determine the upper limit, the curve needs to be redrawn so that blood levels are graphed in ascending rather than descending order and then the point of optimum sensitivity determined. Our ROC curve designated 9 ng/ml as the point of optimum upper limit sensitivity. At 9 ng/ml the false positive responder rate was 33% whereas the true positive responder rate was 83%. Thus our analyses identified a therapeutic range of 4–9 ng/ml, which was significant ($\chi^2 = 7.87$, df = 1,

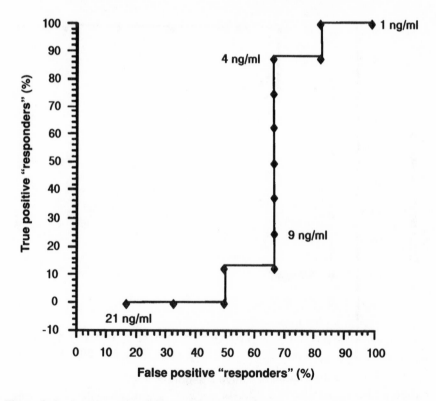

Figure 8–2. Receiver Operating Characteristic (ROC) curve for the relationship between New Haven Schizophrenic Index (NHSI; Astrachan et al. 1972) scores and haloperidol plasma concentrations ranging from 1 to 21 ng/ml for the Garver et al. (1984) data set. True positive "responders," $n = 8$; false positive "responders," $n = 6$.

$P = .005$). The portion of the Figure 8–2 that represents the maximum sensitivity is the area of the graph showing the greatest single precipitous rise in percentage of true positive responders. All six patients with concentrations between 4–9 ng/ml responded to haloperidol. The sensitivity and specificity for haloperidol concentrations of 4–9 ng/ml as a clinical predictor of response were 100% and 75%, respectively.

Linkowski et al. (1984) treated 20 patients who were diagnosed as paranoid schizophrenic according to the RDC. Following a drug wash-out period of greater than 1 week, each patient was treated for 6 weeks with a fixed daily dose of 30 mg of haloperidol. Response was measured at 6 weeks by decline in overall BPRS scores. Fifteen (75%) patients experienced a 30% or greater decline in the BPRS. The authors found no significant relationships between serum haloperidol level and response. Haloperidol plasma levels ranged from 4.3–25.0 ng/ml. As can be seen in Figure 8–3, our ROC curve identified an optimum haloperidol therapeutic effect threshold at 9.5 ng/ml ($\chi^2 = 4.36$, df = 1, $P = .04$). The sensitivity and specificity for this haloperidol blood level as a clinical predictor of response were 87% and 60%, respectively. No upper limit was identified.

Bigelow et al. (1985) treated 19 chronic schizophrenic patients diagnosed according to DSM-III criteria with haloperidol. At the end of a 6-week neuroleptic-free period, the patients were started on a fixed dose of 0.4 mg/kg body weight per day for a minimum of 6 weeks. The BPRS psychosis factor score was used to quantify patient response. Plasma haloperidol concentrations ranged from 6.8 to 29.6 ng/ml. Fourteen (74%) patients experienced a 30% or greater decline in the BPRS psychosis factor. The authors found no significant relationships between serum haloperidol level and the BPRS psychosis factor. Our ROC curve identified 18 ng/ml as the optimum sensitivity point. However, χ^2 analysis found this cutoff point unable to discriminate between responsive and nonresponsive patients ($\chi^2 = 0.42$, df = 1, $P = .52$).

Van Putten et al. (1985) described 34 schizophrenic patients who received fixed doses of haloperidol. The patients had been in a drug-free state for several days to 3 weeks before receiving doses of 5, 10, or 20 mg/day for 4 weeks. At the end of 2 weeks, improvement was measured by the BPRS schizophrenia factor. The data identified 14 (41%) responsive patients who experienced a 30% or greater decline in their score. Like Bigelow et al. (1985), Van Putten et al. (1985) reported no significant correlation between haloperidol blood level and therapeutic response. Blood levels ranged from 0–18.1 ng/ml. Our ROC curve shown in Figure 8–4 identified a lower limit for the blood levels of 2.0 ng/ml. The χ^2 analysis found this cutoff point able to discriminate between responsive and non-responsive patients ($\chi^2 = 6.17$, df = 1, $P = .013$). Despite the finding, its usefulness is dubious because although the specificity was 100%, the sensitivity was only 52%. There was no obvious upper limit for the levels.

Santos et al. (1989) administered fixed doses of haloperidol of 10, 15, or 30 mg/day to 30 schizophrenic patients meeting DSM-III criteria following a wash-out period of at least 10 days. Response was measured as a function of the total BPRS score. Twenty-two (73%) of the patients experienced a 30% or greater decline in their score. The authors found a significant curvilinear relationship between the haloperidol plasma concentrations and the percentage improvement in the total score ($r^2 = .48$) ranging from 12–59 ng/ml. However, the entire relationship was dependent on the existence of a single point. If the point is removed from the data set, the curvi-

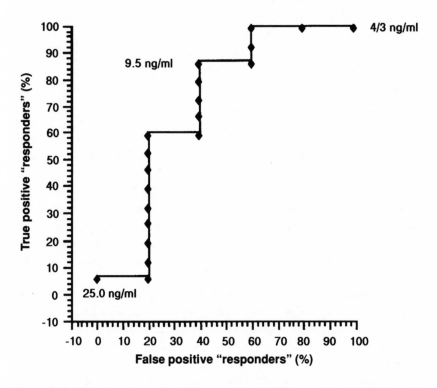

Figure 8–3. Receiver Operating Characteristic (ROC) curve for the relationship between Brief Psychiatric Rating Scale (BPRS; Overall and Gorham 1962) scores and haloperidol plasma concentrations ranging from 4.3 to 25 ng/ml for the Linkowski et al. (1984) data set. True positive "responders," $n = 15$; false positive "responders," $n = 5$.

linear relationship is no longer significant. Instead, the relationship becomes linear. The ROC curve demonstrated the tentativeness of these findings. Our ROC curve (see Figure 8–5), which took into account all data points, identified a lower therapeutic limit of 11 ng/ml (χ^2 = 12.14, df = 1, P = <.0005). The sensitivity and specificity for haloperidol concentrations of 11 ng/ml as a clinical predictor of response were 95% and 64%, respectively. No upper limit is obvious when analyzing these data with ROCs.

Kelly et al. (1990) treated 29 acutely ill schizophrenic patients as defined by DSM-III criteria with fixed doses of haloperidol for a 2-week period. Doses were prospectively adjusted to achieve a haloperidol plasma concentration of either 8–18 ng/ml or 25–35 ng/ml. Response was measured as a function of the total 23-item BPRS score. A 30% decline in total

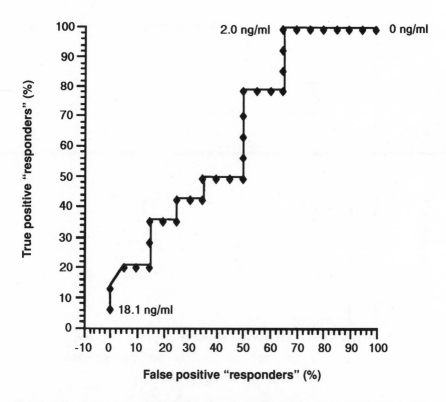

Figure 8–4. Receiver Operating Characteristic (ROC) curve for the relationship between Brief Psychiatric Rating Scale (BPRS; Overall and Gorham 1962) scores and haloperidol plasma concentrations ranging from 0 to 18.1 ng/ml for the Van Putten et al. (1985) data set. True positive "responders," n = 14; false positive "responders," n = 20.

BPRS scores was observed in only 9 (31%) patients. Blood levels ranged from 4.3–52.0 ng/ml. Our ROC curve was unable to demonstrate a lower limit response threshold. However, unlike the other studies, the ROC curve identified an upper limit for the therapeutic effect of haloperidol. As can be seen Figure 8–6, to screen for an upper limit the blood levels are graphed in ascending rather descending order. The upper limit was 15.0 ng/ml ($\chi^2 = 4.58$, df = 1, $P = .03$). The sensitivity and specificity for the upper limit cut-off of 15.0 ng/ml as a clinical predictor of response were 55% and 83%, respectively.

Table 8–2 summarizes the statistical findings regarding these seven relatively well-designed studies. A consistent relationship between haloperidol blood concentrations and clinical response is apparent. The lower limit for

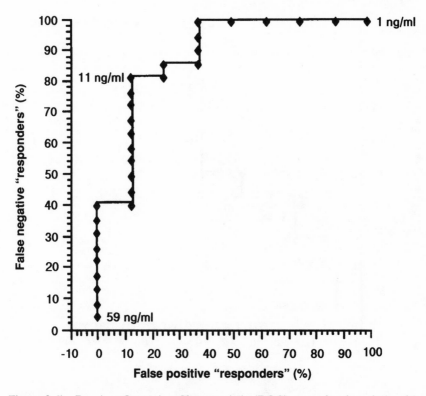

Figure 8–5. Receiver Operating Characteristic (ROC) curve for the relationship between Brief Psychiatric Rating Scale (BPRS; Overall and Gorham 1962) scores and haloperidol plasma concentrations ranging from 1 to 59 ng/ml for the Santos et al. (1989) data set. False negative "responders," $n = 22$; false positive "responders," $n = 8$.

therapeutic effect probably ranges between 5–9.5 ng/ml (Garver et al. 1984; Linkowski et al.1984; Magliozzi et al. 1981; Santos et al. 1989). The upper limit is approximately 14–15 ng/ml (Garver et al. 1984; Kelly et al. 1990). However, some patients will respond outside of this range. This emphasizes the need to use blood level measurements primarily as an adjunct to good clinical care of the patient.

Trifluoperazine

Only one study examined the correlation of trifluoperazine blood levels to therapeutic response. Janicak et al. (1989) studied 36 acutely psychotic patients who met RDC criteria for schizophrenia (30), schizoaffective (5), and

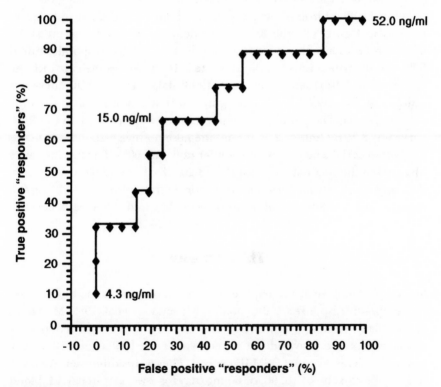

Figure 8–6. Receiver Operating Characteristic (ROC) curve for the relationship between Brief Psychiatric Rating Scale (BPRS; Overall and Gorham 1962) scores and haloperidol plasma concentrations ranging from 4.3 to 52 ng/ml for the Kelly et al. (1990) data set. True positive "responders," $n = 9$; false positive "responders," $n = 20$.

unspecified functional psychosis (1). The patients were drug free for 3 to 36 days before the start of a 2-week fixed-dose course of trifluoperazine at a dose of 10 mg/day. Blood levels ranged from 0.2 to 3.5 ng/ml. At the end of 2 weeks, improvement was measured by the BPRS. Nine (25%) of the patients experienced 25% decrease in their BPRS after 2 weeks. The authors reported a significant curvilinear relationship between trifluoperazine blood level and therapeutic response between 1.05 and 2.25 ng/ml. Our ROC curve identified the same curvilinear relationship limits. The observation was significant (χ^2 = 24.00, df = 1, P = <.0001). The sensitivity and specificity for trifluoperazine concentrations of 1.05–2.25 ng/ml being a clinical predicator of response were 75% and 100%, respectively.

Because of the importance of this positive finding, in contrast to the other studies, the authors were contacted to determine who the nonschizophrenic patients were. The analysis was then repeated using only the data for the 30 schizophrenic patients, of whom 7 were responsive. As can be seen in Figure 8–7, the ROC curve demonstrated 1.05 ng/ml as the lower limit response threshold in which the false positive responder rate is 30% and the true positive responder rate is 100%. As was the case with the Garver et al. (1984) and Kelly et al. (1990) data sets, our ROC curve was redrawn so that blood levels were graphed in ascending rather than descending order. The point of optimum sensitivity determined on the ROC curve was 2.25 ng/ml. At 2.25 ng/ml the false positive responder rate was 83% whereas the true positive responder rate was 100%. The findings were identical to the original analysis (χ^2 = 18.26, df = 1, P = <.0001). The sensitivity and specificity for trifluoperazine concentrations of 1.05–2.25 ng/ml being a clinical predicator of response were 70% and 100%, respectively.

Thiothixene

Several studies have examined the correlation of thiothixene blood levels to therapeutic response (Reifler et al. 1981; Yesavage et al. 1982; Mavroidis et al. 1984a). However, only one of these studies can be regarded as technically acceptable. Mavroidis et al. (1984a) studied 19 acutely ill schizophrenic patients who met DSM-III criteria. They were administered a fixed dose of thiothixene of 16, 30, or 60 mg/day for 2 weeks. On day 14, blood levels ranged from 0.5 to 15.3 ng/ml. At baseline and at 2 weeks, psychopathology was measured by the NHSI. Ten (53%) of the patients experienced a 40% decrease in their NHSI score after 2 weeks. The authors reported a significant curvilinear relationship (r^2 = .35, P < .01) between thiothixene blood level and the percentage decrease in the NHSI. They estimated a therapeutic blood level between 2 to 15 ng/ml. Our ROC curve presented in Figure 8–8, however, identified a threshold therapeutic blood level of 1.7 ng/ml (χ^2 = 4.87, df = 1, P = .027). The sensitivity and specificity for a thiothixene blood level of 1.7 ng/ml as a clinical predictor of response were 86% and 67%, respectively. The curvilinear relationship was entirely dependent on a single patient who had a level of 15.3 ng/ml and who actually demonstrated a 4% increase on the NHSI. If this point is discarded, the relationship is linear rather than curvilinear. However, if it is included in the analysis, the range of 1.7–10.5 ng/ml produced somewhat higher sensitivity and specificity values of 100% and 69%, respectively (χ^2 = 7.89, df = 1, P = .005) than the 1.7 ng/ml lower limit threshold concentration.

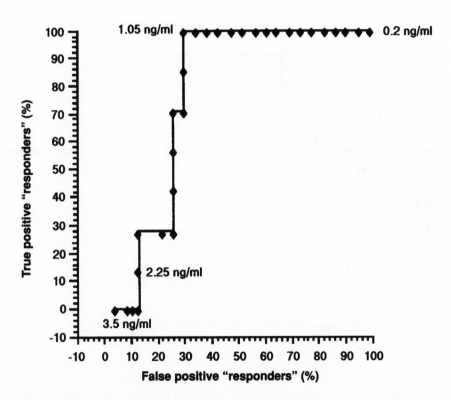

Figure 8–7. Receiver Operating Characteristic (ROC) curve for the relationship between Brief Psychiatric Rating Scale (BPRS; Overall and Gorham 1962) scores and trifluoperazine plasma concentrations ranging from 0.2 to 3.5 ng/ml for the Janicak et al. (1989) data set. True positive "responders," n = 7; false positive "responders," n = 23.

Fluphenazine

Several studies have attempted to discover a correlation between fluphenazine blood levels and therapeutic response. Two have yielded clinically interpretable information. Mavroidis et al. (1984b) examined this relationship in 19 inpatient psychotic schizophrenic patients as defined by DSM-III criteria. A fixed dose of fluphenazine of 5 mg, 10 mg, or 20 mg/day was administered for 2 weeks. Blood drawn on day 14 of the study yielded plasma levels ranging from 0 to 3.2 ng/ml. A significant curvilinear relationship ($n = 19$, $r^2 = .22$, $P < .05$) was reported if the mean blood levels were used. Fluphenazine plasma concentrations between 0.13 and 0.70 ng/ml produced mean improvement of 59% on the NHSI. Patients with

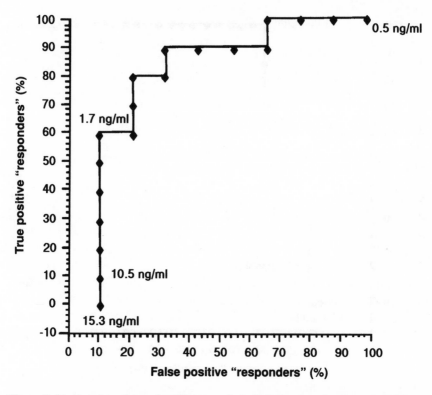

Figure 8–8. Receiver Operating Characteristic (ROC) curve for the relationship between New Haven Schizophrenic Index (NHSI; Astrachan et al. 1972) scores and thiothixene plasma concentrations ranging from 0.5 to 15.3 ng/ml for the Mavroidis et al. (1984) data set. True positive "responders," $n = 10$; false positive "responders," $n = 9$.

blood levels greater than 0.70 ng/ml showed significantly less improvement (mean = 34%).

However, when the fluphenazine concentrations at day 14 were regressed against the percentage change in the NHSI over the 2-week period, the relationship is neither curvilinear nor linear. In fact, if the patient with the highest level at day 14 is removed from the analysis, a much stronger curvilinear relationship is observed ($n = 18$, $r^2 = .48$, $P < .004$). However, the direction of the slope for the curve is inverted. Practically, this means that the patients with the lowest and highest fluphenazine levels experienced the greatest percent decreases in their BPRS scores. Our ROC curve identified a lower therapeutic fluphenazine blood level limit of 2.3 ng/ml. However, this was not significant ($r^2 = .61$, $P = .45$).

Van Putten et al. (1991) studied 72 newly admitted male schizophrenic patients who met DSM-III criteria. They were administered a fixed dose of fluphenazine of 5 mg, 10 mg, or 20 mg/day for 4 weeks. Patients were drug free for at least 3 days before the start of therapy. At baseline and weekly for the next 4 weeks patient improvement was assessed by a variety of measures that included the BPRS and the Clinical Global Impression (CGI) scale (National Institute of Mental Health 1985). Improvement was assessed by logistic regression analysis using the CGI improvement scale and log plasma fluphenazine as the variables. The logistic regression identified a better than 90% probability of response if plasma fluphenazine concentration exceeded approximately 2.7 ng/ml. Interestingly, again using logistic regression analysis, it was found that the maximum percentage (48%) of patients who were rated as "improved without disabling side effects" (e.g., extrapyramidal side effects) occurred at a concentration of 0.67 ng/ml. Additionally, 90% of the patients were predicted to experience disabling side effects at 2.7 ng/ml. Unfortunately, no raw data allowing ROC generation were presented. Thus based on these data, it can tentatively be concluded that a fluphenazine plasma concentration of at least 2–3 ng/ml is most likely to be associated with a response.

Clozapine

Perry et al. (1991) have conducted the only study that attempted to discern a relationship between clozapine and therapeutic response that presented the raw data. It is also the only study that identified a correlation between the drug's plasma concentrations and therapeutic response. Following an 8- to 24-day dose titration phase, 29 inpatients with treatment-resistant schizophrenia (as defined by DSM-III-R criteria) were placed on a fixed clozapine dose of approximately 250 (for 1 patient), 300 (for 3 patients), 350 (for 1 patient), 400 (for 23 patient) or 450 (for 1 patient) mg/day for 4 weeks with blood samples being obtained weekly during this period. Response was defined according to Kane et al.'s criteria (1988) as a 20% or greater change in the total BPRS score from baseline to the end of week 4 of fixed dosing and a final BPRS score of 34 or less.

According to an analysis using the BPRS as the measure of therapeutic effect, a ROC curve demonstrated that the threshold clozapine plasma concentration for therapeutic response was 350 ng/ml. Sixty-four percent of the patients with clozapine plasma concentrations greater than 350 ng/ml responded whereas only 22% of the patients with concentrations less than 350 ng/ml responded. A ROC curve was drawn for all of the clozapine data points. As illustrated in Figure 8–9, a clozapine plasma concentration of 397 ng/ml was the point of maximum sensitivity. Clozapine concentrations of 397 ng/ml or more defined a group of 11 patients that included 7 (64%) of the 11 patients who responded to the drug. The total clozapine concentrations of 509 ng/ml or more defined the same group of 11 patients that included 7 (64%) of the 11 patients who responded to the drug. Thus both drug concentration measurements produced the same degree of sensitivity. Additionally, both drug measurements were able to produce the same degree of specificity. Clozapine concentrations less than 397 ng/ml and total concentrations less than 509 ng/ml predicted nonresponse in 78% (14 of 18) of the patients. Analyses using χ^2 on these data found the differences between the responsive and nonresponsive patients at these particular concentrations significant ($\chi^2 = 4.974$, df = 1, $P = .03$).

Conclusions

At present, neuroleptics differ from tricyclic antidepressants because plasma concentration measurements are not routinely used by most clinicians as a tool to optimize dose adjustment. This is primarily because of a lack of well-designed research supporting the utility of neuroleptic blood concentrations. Also, most laboratories do not routinely perform neuroleptic assays. Of the drugs reviewed, haloperidol, trifluoperazine, thiothixene, and clozapine have been the subjects of well-designed studies that document reasonably consistent relationships between blood concentrations and therapeutic response. Of these, the case for the clinical use of plasma measurements of haloperidol is by far the strongest. Inspection of Table

8–2 indicates that there are four studies that identify a lower limit of 5–9.5 ng/ml and two studies that define 14–15 ng/ml as the upper therapeutic limit. Patients who fail a 6-week trial of haloperidol within this therapeutic range ought to be considered for an alternative agent.

There are only single studies for thiothixene, trifluoperazine, and clozapine that document a correlation between therapeutic response and blood level. Based on sample size considerations and our analyses it seems logical that the next drug of choice would be trifluoperazine (1.05–2.25 ng/ml) if the patient is not considered treatment refractory. However, if the patient is treatment refractory, clozapine (397 ng/ml or more) would be the only treatment of choice remaining for the patient.

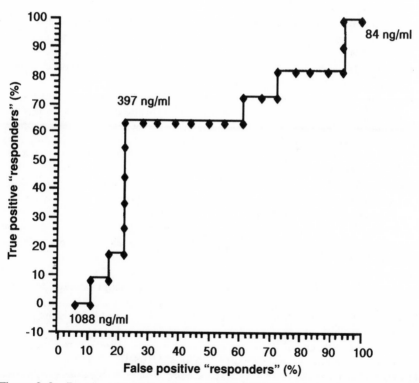

Figure 8–9. Receiver Operating Characteristic (ROC) curve for the relationship between Brief Psychiatric Rating Scale (BPRS; Overall and Gorham 1962) scores and clozapine plasma concentrations ranging from 84 to 1,088 ng/ml for the Perry et al. (1991) data set. True positive "responders," $n = 11$; false positive "responders," $n = 18$.

References

American Psychiatric Association: Diagnostic and Statistical Manual of Mental Disorders, 3rd Edition. Washington, DC, American Psychiatric Association, 1980

American Psychiatric Association: Diagnostic and Statistical Manual of Mental Disorders, 3rd Edition, Revised. Washington, DC, American Psychiatric Association, 1987

Asberg M, Perris C, Schalling D, et al: A comprehensive psychiatric rating scale. Acta Psychiatr Scand Suppl 271:5–27, 1978

Astrachan BM, Harrow M, Adler D, et al: A checklist for the diagnosis of schizophrenia. Br J Psychiatry 121:529–539, 1972

Bigelow LB, Krich DG, Braun T, et al: Absence of relationship of serum haloperidol concentration and clinical response in chronic schizophrenia: a fixed-dose study: Psychopharmacol Bull 21:66–68, 1985

Dahl SG: Plasma level monitoring of antipsychotic drugs: clinical utility. Clin Pharmacokinet 11:36–61, 1986

Garver DL, Hirschowitz J, Glicksteen GA, et al: Haloperidol plasma and red blood cell levels and clinical antipsychotic response. J Clin Psychopharmacol 4:133–137, 1984

Janicak PG, Javaid JI, Sharma RP, et al: Trifluoperazine plasma levels and clinical response. J Clin Psychopharmacol 9:340–346, 1989

Kane J, Honigfeld G, Singer J, et al: Clozapine for the treatment-resistant schizophrenic. A double-blind comparison with chlorpromazine. Arch Gen Psychiatry 45:489–496, 1988

Kelly MW, Perry PJ, Coryell WH, et al: Reduced haloperidol plasma concentration and clinical response in acute exacerbations of schizophrenia. Psychopharmacology (Berl) 102:514–520, 1990

Levinson DF, Simpson GM, Singh H, et al: Neuroleptic plasma level may predict response in patients who meet a criterion for improvement (letter). Arch Gen Psychiatry 45:877–879, 1988

Linkowski P, Hubain P, von Frenckell R, et al: Haloperidol plasma levels and clinical response in paranoid schizophrenics. Eur Arch Psychiatry Neurol Sci 234:231–236, 1984

Magliozzi JR, Hollister LE, Arnold KV, et al: Relationship of serum haloperidol levels to clinical response in schizophrenic patients. Am J Psychiatry 138:365–367, 1981

Mavroidis ML, Kanter J, Hirschowitz, et al: Clinical relevance of thiothixene plasma levels. J Clin Psychopharmacol 4:155–157, 1984a

Mavroidis ML, Kanter DR, Hirschowitz J, et al: Fluphenazine plasma levels and clinical response. J Clin Psychiatry 45:370–373, 1984b

Mossman D, Somoza E: ROC curves, test accuracy, and the description of diagnostic tests. Journal of Neuropsychiatry and Clinical Neuroscience 3:330–333, 1991

National Institute of Mental Health: CGI (Clinical Global Impression) Scale. Psychopharmacol Bull 21:839–843, 1985

Overall JE, Gorham DR: The Brief Psychiatric Rating Scale. Psychol Rep 10:799–812, 1962

Perry PJ, Miller DD, Arndt SV, et al: Clozapine and norclozapine plasma concentrations and clinical response of treatment-refractory schizophrenic patients. Am J Psychiatry 148:231–235, 1991

Reifler BV, Ward N, Davis CM, et al: Thiothixene plasma levels and clinical response in acute schizophrenia. J Clin Psychiatry 42:207–211, 1981

Santos JL, Cabranes JA, Vazquez C: Clinical response and plasma haloperidol levels in chronic and subchronic schizophrenia. Biol Psychiatry 26:381–388, 1989

Spitzer RL, Endicott J, Robins E: Research diagnostic criteria: rationale and reliability. Arch Gen Psychiatry 35:773–782, 1978

Van Putten T, May PRA, Jenden DJ, et al: Does a plasma level of chlorpromazine help? Psychol Med 11:729–734, 1981

Van Putten T, Marder SR, May PRA, et al: Plasma level of haloperidol and clinical response. Psychopharmacol Bull 21:69–72, 1985

Van Putten T, Aravagiri M, Marder SR, et al: Plasma fluphenazine levels and clinical response in newly admitted schizophrenic patients. Psychopharmacol Bull 27:91–96, 1991

Wode-Helgodt B, Borg S, Fyro B, et al: Clinical effects and drug concentrations in plasma and cerebrospinal fluid in psychotic patients treated with fixed doses of chlorpromazine. Acta Psychiatr Scand 58:149–173, 1978

Yesavage JA, Becker J, Werner PD, et al: Serum level monitoring of thiothixene in schizophrenia: acute single-dose levels at fixed doses. Am J Psychiatry 139:174–178, 1982

Use and Interpretation of Neuroleptic Plasma Levels

Stephen R. Marder, M.D.
John M. Davis, M.D.
Philip G. Janicak, M.D.

T he authors in this book have presented a number of viewpoints about the clinical value of neuroleptic plasma concentrations. Although there are marked differences among the cited studies, there are also consistent patterns that have developed in recent years. As a result, we believe that this is an appropriate time to review those circumstances in which neuroleptic plasma levels may be clinically useful.

Measurement of Plasma Levels on a Routine Basis

Approximately three out of four acutely ill, schizophrenic patients will demonstrate substantial improvement when they are administered a moderate dose of an antipsychotic medication. This dose is usually between 300 and 1,000 mg of chlorpromazine, 5 and 20 mg of haloperidol, or 5 and 20 mg of fluphenazine daily (Baldessarini et al. 1988). If patients demonstrate substantial clinical improvement after a month or less with drug treatment, there is little likelihood that a plasma level measurement will add any significant information. As noted in Chapters 1, 2, and 3, the correlations between plasma level and clinical response are relatively low and may not add significantly to the information about a given patient's drug dose. Moreover, most patients given doses in the above range will also have plasma levels in the putative therapeutic ranges.

The reasons for relatively weak correlations between plasma levels and clinical response are discussed in Chapter 1 by Cohen and Waternaux, who point out that "tissue sensitivity" in addition to drug levels probably play an important role in determining response. This phenomenon is most evident for drug side effects where, for example, one patient may experience tormenting akathisia at levels that are easily tolerated by others. In addition, drug plasma levels may not reflect drug levels in the brain, which may be affected by differences in protein binding, drug metabolism, passage across the blood-brain barrier, and other factors. Finally, there are schizophrenic patients who are poorly responsive to neuroleptics regardless of the level. As a result, studies of relationships between plasma levels and clinical response tend to find a wide range of responses at almost every level of drug, with the possible exception of subtherapeutic levels. After discussing the major limitations of neuroleptic plasma levels in clinical practice, we review those selected circumstances where they may be helpful.

Patients Who Respond Poorly to Oral Antipsychotics

Plasma level measurement may have a role in individuals who have received adequate antipsychotic doses but remain severely symptomatic. If the patient has been treated with one of the drugs for which there are adequate data, such as haloperidol, fluphenazine, trifluoperazine, thiothixene, or perphenazine, a low plasma concentration may explain an inadequate response. For example, patient noncompliance or partial compliance occurs frequently in both inpatient and outpatient settings. Moreover, noncompliance can be surreptitious and therefore inaccessible to a clinical examination.

Low plasma concentrations may also be evidence of poor drug absorption or accelerated metabolism (reviewed in Van Putten et al. 1991a). Nearly every study of antipsychotic plasma concentrations has found that individuals demonstrate wide variations in plasma concentrations when they are administered the same drug dose. Although it makes intuitive sense that these differences in plasma concentrations are related to clinical response, the evidence supporting a relationship between a poor outcome and unusual metabolism rests on a small number of cases. In addition, there are relatively few cases from controlled studies of individual poorly responding patients who had plasma levels below the putative therapeutic threshold. Data from a number of studies (reviewed in this book by Janicak,

Davis, Van Putten, and Levinson) suggest increasing the dose in a non-responsive patient who has a low plasma level (for example, < 5 ng/ml of haloperidol, 1 ng/ml of trifluoperazine, or 1 ng/ml of fluphenazine). At this stage, more data on plasma concentrations of clozapine would be helpful. Generally, when plasma levels are below the range generally seen clinically, the physician should consider raising the dose.

Other Drug Interactions With Antipsychotics

A number of drugs can influence antipsychotic plasma levels as a result of their effects on drug metabolism. Examples include certain heterocyclic antidepressants, fluoxetine, beta blockers, and cimetidine, all of which may increase plasma levels by competing for enzyme-binding sites. Conversely, barbiturates and carbamazepine may decrease plasma levels by enhancing metabolism of the neuroleptic. For example, studies indicate that carbamazepine can reduce plasma levels of haloperidol by 50% (Jann et al. 1985). Therefore, when clinicians are combining a neuroleptic with a drug likely to alter pharmacokinetics, plasma level monitoring may provide useful information. In the very young, the elderly, and the medically compromised, the pharmacokinetics of neuroleptics may be significantly altered and may require plasma level measurements to assure adequate levels and avoid toxicity.

Patients Experiencing Side Effects

Side effects such as mild akathisia or akinesia can be difficult to diagnose, particularly in patients who are inarticulate or uncommunicative. Akathisia, in particular, can often present as anxiety and/or agitation. As a result, clinicians are commonly faced with the following dilemma: is the patient failing to recover from a psychotic episode because of side effects associated with too high a drug dose or persistence of psychotic symptoms because of an insufficient dose?

As discussed in Chapter 1, the relationship between side effects and plasma level may be stronger than the relationship between clinical response and plasma level. Therefore, a relatively high level (e.g. >15–25 ng/ml of haloperidol, 2.5 ng/ml of fluphenazine, or 2.3 ng/ml of trifluoperazine) might dictate a dose reduction. This may explain the results described in Chapter 4: where patients with relatively high haloperidol plasma levels (i.e., >12 ng/ml) improved when their dose was decreased.

Plasma Level Monitoring in Maintenance Therapy

A serious drawback in maintenance therapy is that clinical response cannot be monitored against drug dose, as patients are usually stable when decisions about dose adjustment are made. Recent studies have pointed to the importance of using as low a maintenance dose as possible to minimize adverse effects while still preventing a relapse. Chapter 7 suggests that plasma level measurements may help clinicians safely reduce maintenances doses. They found that relatively low fluphenazine plasma levels (i.e., < 0.8 ng/ml) were associated with an increased risk of relapse, and that a relatively small dose (and presumably plasma level) increase may substantially decrease this risk. However, until this is confirmed, we believe there is insufficient data to recommend the *routine* use of plasma levels for long-term maintenance.

Despite these limited data, however, there may be situations where clinicians would benefit from measuring plasma concentrations in maintenance therapy. For example, if patients have relapsed on several occasions despite receiving what seems to be a reasonable drug dose, a plasma level measurement may be indicated. If the plasma level is low and the patient is receiving an oral preparation, poor compliance should be considered. Switching to a long-acting depot form may be helpful in these circumstances. Similarly, a low plasma level on an oral or depot preparation suggests that raising the dose is a reasonable intervention. For patients who have a high risk associated with relapse (e.g., those who make serious suicide attempts or become violent), a plasma level that is in the therapeutic range for fluphenazine or haloperidol may increase the margin of safety. For patients whose dose is limited by side effects, a plasma level measurement may help to assure the clinician that the individual is receiving an adequate dose.

Usefulness of Individual Drugs

As mentioned in Chapter 2, therapeutic ranges should be established for individual drugs, as well as for different illnesses. Variations in side-effect profiles, drug metabolism, or route of administration will dictate the usefulness of plasma levels. Moreover, there are some drugs (e.g., clozapine) for which plasma level measurements will probably be unavailable to the clinician. Other drug plasma level measurements, such as fluphenazine, may be available, but the analytical methods can lack the sensitivity required to measure very low levels.

Because the most information is available for haloperidol, a number of studies reviewed or described in this book have focused on the relationship between clinical effect and haloperidol plasma levels. Although not all studies found a clinically relevant relationship, overall a convincing pattern has emerged. As previously mentioned, patients unresponsive to a trial with haloperidol, when plasma levels are below 5 ng/ml, may benefit from an dose *increase.* Similarly, those patients with plasma levels greater than 15–18 ng/ml may benefit from a dose *decrease.* In addition, as noted in Chapter 2, plasma concentrations can be used to establish the adequacy of pharmacotherapy in nonresponsive patients. Therefore, when patients have not responded to 4 to 6 weeks of haloperidol with a plasma level in the proposed therapeutic range, it is probably appropriate to change to another antipsychotic.

Although the usefulness of plasma levels for other neuroleptics is not as well established, as noted in Chapter 3, there are studies that suggest that measurements of plasma fluphenazine may also be useful. Their findings, as well as similar findings by Van Putten et al. (1991b) indicate that plasma levels in the range of 1–2 ng/ml are likely to be effective. As noted in Chapter 2, evidence indicates that for trifluoperazine, plasma levels in the range of 1–2 ng/ml also appear to be most effective. Studies by Bolvig-Hansen and Larsen (1985), Janicak et al. (1989), and Mazure et al. (1990) suggest that a range of 0.8–2.4 ng/ml for perphenazine might be effective. Additional information will be needed before making recommendations for other drugs. Nevertheless, a number of studies are available that may be informative to clinicians.

Medical-Legal Situations

There may also be a role for monitoring the adequacy of neuroleptic drug therapy in some patients who may be at risk for violent behavior (self or other directed) when not properly medicated. Plasma levels could play a role in both monitoring compliance and assuring the legal system that maximum efforts have been devoted to preventing relapse.

References

Baldessarini RJ, Cohen BM, Teicher MH: Significance of neuroleptic dose and plasma level in the pharmacological treatment of psychoses. Arch Gen Psychiatry 45:79–90, 1988

Bolvig-Hansen L, Larsen NE: Therapeutic advantages of monitoring plasma concentrations of perphenazine in clinical practice. Psychopharmacology (Berl) 87:16–19, 1985

Janicak PG, Javaid JI, Sharma RP, et al: Trifluoperazine plasma levels and clinical response. J Clin Psychopharmacol 9:340–346, 1989

Jann MW, Ereshefsky l, Sakalad SR: Effects of carbamezepine on plasma haloperidol levels. J Clin Psychopharmacol 5:106–109, 1985

Mazure CM, Nelson JC, Jatlow PI, et al:The relationship between perphenazine levels, early resolution of psychotic symptoms, and side effects. J Clin Psychiatry 51:335–339. 1990

Van Putten T, Marder SR, Wirshing WC, et al: Neuroleptic plasma levels. Schizophr Bull 17:197–216, 1991a

Van Putten T, Aravagiri M, Marder S, et al: Plasma fluphenazine levels and clinical response in newly admitted schizophrenic patients. Psychopharmacol Bull 27:91–96, 1991b

Index

Page numbers in **boldface** *type refer to tables or figures.*

Absorption of drugs, 1, 11, 19
definition of, **21**
individual differences in, 2
for oral vs. depot drugs, 104
in poor responders to oral
drugs, 138
Administration route
bioavailability related to, 19
depot drugs, 101–111
poor "responders" to oral drugs,
138–139
Agitation, 139
Akathisia, 138, 139
fluphenazine-induced, 53, **54**,
57, 58
haloperidol-induced, 72
Amobarbital sodium, 50
Anesthesia, 18
Antidepressants, 23, 132
interaction with neuroleptics,
139
monitoring plasma levels of, 17
Antipsychotics. *See* Neuroleptics
Anxiety, 139
Assay methods, 22–23, **23–25**, 114,
116–117
biological vs. chemical, 23,
24–25
blood collection and handling
methods, 23
gas chromatography-mass
spectrometry, **24**

gas-liquid chromatography, 23,
23–24
high-performance liquid
chromatography, 23, **24**
radioimmunoassay, **25**
radioreceptor assays, 23, **23**, **25**
sensitivity of, 46–47, 103–104
spectrometric, **24**

Barbiturates, 139
Benztropine mesylate
fluphenazine and, 50, **54**
haloperidol and, 79
Beta blockers, 139
Bioavailability, 19
related to administration route,
19, 104
Biological half-life ($t_{1/2}$), 19, **21**
Blood-brain barrier, 138
Blood collection and handling
methods, 23
Bradykinesia, 72
Brain levels of neuroleptics, 2, 8–10
Brief Psychiatric Rating Scale
(BPRS), 104, 114, **116–117**
for patients in chlorpromazine
study, 119
for patients in clozapine studies,
87–91, **88**, **91–92**, **96**, 132,
133
for patients in fluphenazine
studies, 50, **52**, 131

Brief Psychiatric Rating Scale
(BPRS) *(continued)*
  for patients in haloperidol
    studies, **30**, 31–33, 65–69,
    67–69, 79–81, **80**, 120, **121**,
    124–127
  for patients in trifluoperazine
    studies, **29**, 128, **129**
Butaperazine, 27
  fixed-dose studies of correlation
    of plasma level and clinical
    response to, **5**
  plasma levels by gas-liquid
    chromatography and
    radioreceptor assays, **23**
Butyrophenone metabolism, 11

Carbamazepine
  interaction with neuroleptics,
    72, 139
  monitoring plasma levels of, 17
Cerebrospinal fluid (CSF) drug
    concentration, 114
  of chlorpromazine, 119
"Chemical restraint," 73
Chloral hydrate, 50
Chlorpromazine
  bioavailability related to
    administration route, 19
  dosage of, **5**, 10, 27, 137
  efficacy of
    compared with fluphenazine,
      45
    at high plasma levels, 78
  fixed-dose studies of correlation
    of plasma level and clinical
    response to, **5**, 77
  metabolites of, 21
  methodological problems in
    studies of, 46

occupancy of D_2-receptors in
    brain, 9, **9**
  plasma levels of, 26–27
  sensitivity and specificity of
    plasma levels for predicting
    response to, 115, 119–120
Chlorpromazine sulfoxide, 21
Cimetidine, 139
Clearance (Cl), 19
  definition of, **21**
Clinical effects of drugs. *See*
    Therapeutic effects of drugs
Clinical Global Impression (CGI)
    Scale
  for patients in fluphenazine
    study, 131
  for patients in haloperidol
    studies, **30**, 31–32, **70**, 72,
    79–81, **80**
Clozapine, 85–98
  action on dopamine receptors,
    9, 9–10, 85
  availability of, 111
  Brief Psychiatric Rating Scale
    response to, **88**, 89–91,
    91–92, **96**, 97
    anergia factor, 90, 97
    interpersonal disturbance
      factor, 90
    thought disturbance factor,
      90
  clinical response related to
    plasma levels of, 85–87, **88**
  dosage for "responders" and
    "nonresponders" to, 87
  efficacy of, 85
  mechanism of action of, 85
  optimal plasma level for
    treatment-resistant patients,
    97, 98

Receiver Operating
    Characteristic curves for,
    87–89, **91–95**
    Brief Psychiatric Rating Scale
        response, 90–91, **91–92**
    Scale for Assessment of
        Negative Symptoms
        response, 91–98, **94–95**
    Scale for Assessment of
        Positive Symptoms
        response, 91–98, **93, 95**
    sedation due to, 87
    sensitivity and specificity of
        plasma levels for predicting
        response to, 90–98, **118**,
        131–132, **133**
Cogentin. *See* Benztropine mesylate
Comprehensive
    Psychopathological Rating
    Scale (CPRS), 119

Depot neuroleptics, 101–111. *See
    also* specific drugs
    benefits of monitoring plasma
        levels of, 101–102
    for maintenance therapy, 101
    pharmacokinetics compared
        with oral drugs, 104
    plasma levels of fluphenazine
        decanoate, 27, 28, 46, 48, 57,
        102, **103**, 105–110, **107–109**
    plasma levels of haloperidol
        decanoate, 110
    problems in studying plasma
        levels of, 102–105
    assay sensitivity, 103–104
    measurement of side effects,
        104–105
    metabolism of oral vs. depot
        drugs, 104

    noncompliance, 105
    outcome measurement, 104
    time to reach steady-state
        level, 102–103, **103**
Desmethylclozapine, 87
N-Didesmethylchlorpromazine, 21
Distribution of drugs, 1, 19
    blood-to-brain distribution
        ratios, 114
    factors causing individual
        differences in, 2
    metabolites, 3
    volume of distribution defined,
        21
Dopamine receptors
    clozapine actions on, 85
    neuroleptic mediation by D_3-,
        D_4-, and D_5-receptors, 9
    neuroleptic occupancy of
        D_2-receptors, **9**, 9–10
Dose, 137
    adjustments of
        according to clinical response,
            18, 22
        formula to achieve targeted
            steady-state concentration,
            34, **35**
        trial-and-error, 2
    of chlorpromazine, 27
    for clinical trials of clinical
        effects related to plasma
        levels, **5**, 10
    correlation with side effects, 8
    D_2-receptor occupancy and, 10
    establishing minimally effective
        dose, 18
    fixed-dose studies of drug
        effects, 4, 22
    of fluphenazine decanoate,
        108–109

Dose *(continued)*
of haloperidol, 71, **71**
for maintenance therapy, 101
of perphenazine, 28
of phenothiazines for elderly
patients, 11
reduction of, 10, 11
related to side effects, 139–140
related to therapeutic effects of
drugs, 2
strategy for, 22
therapeutic window and, 19, **20**
of thiothixene, 28
of trifluoperazine, 29
Drug interactions, 139
with haloperidol, 72

Elderly patients
metabolism and side effects of
phenothiazines in, 11
pharmacokinetics in, 139
Elimination of drugs, 1
elimination rate constant
defined, **21**
primary route of, 19
Extrapyramidal symptoms. *See also*
Side effects
fluphenazine-induced, 53, **54**,
57, 58
haloperidol-induced, 72–73, **73**
in patients who metabolize
debrisoquine poorly, 71

First-pass effect, 19, 104
definition of, **21**
Fluoxetine, 139
Fluphenazine, 45–58
acute treatment studies of
plasma levels of, 47–48

benefits of measuring plasma
levels of, 57–58
dosage of, 137
efficacy related to, 45–46, 57
high dose, 46
increasing dose in patients
with low plasma level, 139
low-to-moderate dose, 46
original studies of, 45
related to side effects, 139
efficacy studies of, 45–46
compared with other
neuroleptics, 45
extrapyramidal symptoms
related to dose and plasma
levels of, 53, **54**, 57, 58
fixed-dose studies of correlation
of plasma level and clinical
response to, **5**
gas-liquid chromatography and
radioreceptor assays of
plasma levels of, **23**, 46–48
history of, 45
maximal symptom reduction
related to plasma levels of, 57
metabolism of, 104
metabolites of, 56
methodological problems in
studies of, 46
occupancy of D_2-receptors in
brain, **9**
outcome prediction based on
dose and plasma levels of,
53, 56–57
plasma levels of, 27–28
"rapid neuroleptization" with,
46
sensitivity and specificity of
plasma levels for predicting
response to, **118**, 130–131

study of plasma levels during
    acute treatment, 49–58, 50
discussion of, 53–58
dropouts from, 50
drugs given concurrently with,
    50
excluding treatment-resistant
    patients from, 55
methods and procedure for,
    50–51
results of, 51–53, **52, 54**
setting for, 49
subjects for, 49–50
therapeutic window for, 27, 47–48
Fluphenazine decanoate, 27, 28,
    46, 48, 57
problems in studying plasma
    levels of, 102–104
assay sensitivity, 103–104
time to reach steady-state
    level, 102, **103**
studies of plasma levels of,
    105–110, **107–109**
assay method for, 106
blood sampling schedule for,
    106
clinical benefits of, 109–110
compared with studies of oral
    fluphenazine, 107–108
optimal dose indicated by,
    108–109
related to neurological side
    effects, 106–107
related to psychotic
    exacerbation risk, 106,
    107–109
subjects for, 105

Gas chromatography-mass
    spectrometry (GC-MS), **24**

Gas-liquid chromatography
    (GLC), 23, **23–24**, **30**, 31, 114,
    116–117
sensitivity of, 46
Global Assessment Scale (GAS), **29**

Haldol. *See* Haloperidol
Haloperidol, 63–73, 77–82
bioavailability related to
    administration route, 19
clinical state of patients with
    toxic plasma levels of, 65,
    69–70
dosage of, **5**, 10, 137
correlation with plasma levels,
    71, **71**
increasing dose in patients
    with low plasma level, 139
related to side effects, 139–140
drug interactions with, 72
elimination in poor
    debrisoquine metabolizers,
    71
fixed-dose studies of correlation
    of plasma level and clinical
    response to, **5–6**, 6, 63–65, **64**
gas-liquid chromatography and
    radioreceptor assays of
    plasma levels of, **23**
Illinois study of, 79–82
discussion of, 81–82
dosage schedules for, 79
informed consent for, 79
methods of, 79–80
results of, **80**, 80–81
subjects for, 79
metabolite of, 21, 29–30
occupancy of D_2-receptors in
    brain, 9, **9**
plasma levels of, 29–33, **30**

Haloperidol *(continued)*
  measured by "index of
    improvement," 32
  predicting outcome based on,
    71, 141
  plateau relationship for, 63
  Receiver Operating
    Characteristic curves for,
    120–127, **121–122**, **124–127**
  reduced, 21, 29–30
  sensitivity and specificity of
    plasma levels for predicting
    response to, **118**
  side effects of, 72–73, **73**
  therapeutic window for, **30**,
    30–33, 63–65, **64**, 69
  used for "chemical restraint," 73
  use of high plasma levels in
    neuroleptic-resistant
    patients, 66
  Van Putten study of, 66–73
    discussion of, 69–73
    raising plasma levels in
      relatively nonresponsive
      patients in, 68–69, **69**
    reducing excessive plasma
      levels in, 67–72, **68**
    results of, 66–67, **67**
    subjects for, 66
Haloperidol decanoate, 110
  time to reach steady-state level,
    102
Helmert contrast, 80–81
High-performance liquid
  chromatography (HPLC), 23,
  24, 47, 114, **116–117**
7-Hydroxy-chlorpromazine, 21
7-Hydroxy-*N*-didesmethylchlorprom
  azine, 21
7-Hydroxyfluphenazine, 105

Lithium, 17
Long-acting injectable
  neuroleptics (LINs). *See* Depot
  neuroleptics
Long-term drug effects, 3

Maintenance therapy. *See also*
  Depot neuroleptics
  benefits of monitoring plasma
    levels in, 101–102, 110–111,
    140
  depot neuroleptics for, 101–111
  problems in studying plasma
    levels in, 102–105, 140
Medical-legal situations, 141
Metabolism of drugs, 1, 11, 19, 138
  individual differences in, 2
  in older vs. younger patients, 11
  for oral vs. depot drugs, 104
  in poor "responders" to oral
    drugs, 138
Metabolites, 2–3
  of chlorpromazine, 21
  clinically active, 19–21
  of fluphenazine, 56
  of haloperidol, 21, 29–30
  of trifluoperazine, 28–29
Methodological issues, 21–26
  affecting preliminary results of
    targeted study design, 33–39
  assay methods, 22–23, **23–25**
  dose strategy, 22, 78
  patient population, 26, 78
  requirements for clinical studies,
    3–4, 78
  study design, 26
  types of, 21

Neuroleptic malignant syndrome,
  26

Neuroleptic plasma levels
  benefits of monitoring, 113
  clinical usefulness of, 10–11
  correlation with drug effects, 1–8
  drugs monitored by, 17
  indications for measurement of,
    11, 39
  limitations and values of, 1–11
  monitoring in maintenance
    therapy, 101–111, 140
  preliminary results of targeted
    study of, 33–39
    achieving targeted steady-state
      drug concentration, 34, **35**
    high group, 35, **38**, 39
    identification of drug
      "responders" and
      "nonresponders," 35
    low group, 35, **36**
    middle group, 35, **37**, 39
  problems in interpretation of, 2–3
  role for monitoring in
    medical-legal situations, 141
  routine measurement of,
    137–138
  sensitivity and specificity as
    predictor of response,
    90–98, 113–133
  of specific drugs
    butaperazine, 27
    chlorpromazine, 26–27
    clozapine, 85–98
    fluphenazine, 27–28, 45–58
    haloperidol, 29–33, **30**, 63–73,
      77–82
    perphenazine, 28
    thiothixene, 28
    trifluoperazine, 28–29, **29**
  theoretical basis for monitoring
    of, 18–21

usefulness for individual drugs,
    140–141
  variations related to metabolic
    rate, 39
Neuroleptics
  atypical. *See* Clozapine
  blood-to-brain distribution ratios
    for, 114
  drug interactions with, 139
  half-life to response with, 18
  levels at active sites in brain,
    8–10, **9**
  long-acting injectable (LINs),
    101–111. *See also* Depot
    neuroleptics
  poor responders to oral drugs,
    138–139
  protein binding of, 2, 114, 130
  rate of response to, 137
  sites of concentration of, 2
New Haven Schizophrenic Index
    (NHSI), 114, **117**
  for patients in fluphenazine
    studies, 47, 48, 130–131
  for patients in haloperidol study,
    30, 30–31, 121
  for patients in thiothixene study,
    128–129, **130**
Noncompliance, 11, 39, 58, 105,
    113, 138
α_1-Noradrenergic receptors, 9
Norclozapine, 87, 90, 93, 95
Nurses' Observation Scale for
    Inpatient Evaluation (NOSIE),
    32

Patient population, 26
Perphenazine, 28
  dose of, 28

Perphenazine *(continued)*
  fixed-dose studies of correlation
    of plasma level and clinical
    response to, **5**
  occupancy of D$_2$-receptors in
    brain, **9**
Pharmacokinetics, 19
  clinical, 19
  definition of, 19
  drug interactions affecting, 139
  factors in, **21**
  of oral vs. depot neuroleptics,
    104
Phenothiazines. *See also* specific
    drugs
  blood collection and handling
    for measurement of, 23
  metabolism and side effects in
    elderly patients, 11
Positron-emission tomography
    (PET), 9
Protein binding, 2, 114, 138

Radioimmunoassay (RIA), **16–117**,
    25, **30**, 31–32, 47, 114
  of fluphenazine levels, 47, 48,
    50, 58, 102, 106
Radioreceptor assays (RRA), 23,
    23, **25**, **30**, 31, 46, 114
  disadvantages of, 114
  of fluphenazine levels, 48
Receiver Operating Characteristic
    (ROC) curves, 113–115, **118**
  construction of, 114–115
  graphing of data points on, 115
  identifying optimum sensitivity
    point on, 115
  rates of data on, 115
  for specific drugs

clozapine, 87–89, **91–95**, 132,
    133
haloperidol, 120–127,
    121–122, **124–127**
thiothixene, 128–129, **130**
trifluoperazine, 127–128, **129**
Research Diagnostic Criteria
    (RDC), 31, 47, 49, 79, 114,
    116–117
Reserpine, 45
Response to drugs. *See also*
    Therapeutic effects of drugs
  changes over time in, 3
  dose adjustments based on, 18,
    22
  failure of, 26
  individual differences in, 3

Scale for Assessment of Negative
    Symptoms (SANS)
  for patients in clozapine study,
    87, **88**, 91–98, **94–96**
  for patients in fluphenazine
    study, 50, 51
Scale for Assessment of Positive
    Symptoms (SAPS), for patients
    in clozapine study, 87, **88**,
    91–98, **93**, **95–96**
Schedule for Affective Disorders
    and Schizophrenia (SADS), 49
Schizoaffective disorder
  chlorpromazine for, 119
  clozapine for, 86
  fluphenazine for, 49
  haloperidol for, 65
Sensitivity and specificity of
    neuroleptic plasma levels,
    113–133
  characteristics of studies of,
    116–117

conclusions about, 132–133
criteria for inclusion in analysis
of, 113–114
Receiver Operating
Characteristic curves of,
113–115, **118**
for specific drugs
chlorpromazine, 115, 119–120
clozapine, 90–98, **118**,
131–132, **133**
fluphenazine, **118**, 130–131
haloperidol, **118**, 120–127,
121–122, 124–127
thiothixene, **118**, 128–129, **130**
trifluoperazine, **118**, 127–128,
129
Sensitivity of drug assays, 46–47,
103–104
Serotonin (5-HT$_2$) receptor, 9
Side effects, 138, 139–140. *See also*
Extrapyramidal symptoms
correlation with plasma levels
and dose, 8, 19
delayed, 1–2
dose related to, 139–140
of fluphenazine decanoate,
106–107
of haloperidol, 72–73, **73**
measuring for maintenance
therapy, 104–105
monitoring of, 11
Simpson-Angus Scale, 65
Simpson Neurological Rating
Scale (NRS), 50, 51, **54**
Simpson Tardive Dyskinesia Rating
Scale (TDRS), 50
Spectrometric techniques, **24**
Steady-state concentration (C$_{SS}$),
defined, **21**
Study design, 3–4, 26

Tardive dyskinesia, 1, 26
Tardive dystonia, 26
Therapeutic effects of drugs
correlation with blood levels,
1–8, 10–11
for butaperazine, 27
for chlorpromazine, 26–27
clinical studies of, 4–8, **5–7**
for fluphenazine, 27–28
for haloperidol, 29–33, **30**
methodological requirements
for study of, 3–4
for perphenazine, 28
results of studies of, 6–8, **6–7**
sensitivity and specificity of,
113–133
side effects and, 8
for thiothixene, 28
for trifluoperazine, 28–29, **29**
long-term, 3
time to develop, 1, 3, 18
Therapeutic window, 19, **20**, 39, 78
for fluphenazine, 27, 47–48
for haloperidol, **30**, 30–33,
63–65, **64**, 69
missing lower end of, 22
for trifluoperazine, 28–29
Thioridazine
efficacy compared with
fluphenazine, 45
fixed-dose studies of correlation
of plasma level and clinical
response to, **5**, 6–7, **7**
occupancy of D$_2$-receptors in
brain, **9**
Thiothixene, 28
dose of, 28
fixed-dose studies of correlation
of plasma level and clinical
response to, **5**

Thiothixene *(continued)*
  sensitivity and specificity of
    plasma levels for predicting
    response to, **118**, 128–129,
    130
Treatment-resistant patients, 26
  clozapine for, 85
  fluphenazine for, 55
Trifluoperazine, 28–29, **29**
  dose of, 29
    increasing dose in patients
      with low plasma level, 139
    related to side effects, 139
    fixed-dose studies of correlation
      of plasma level and clinical
      response to, **5**

  metabolites of, 28–29
  plasma levels by gas-liquid
    chromatography and
    radioreceptor assays, **23**
  sensitivity and specificity of
    plasma levels for predicting
    response to, **118**, 127–128,
    129
  therapeutic window for, 28–29

Urinary excretion of drugs, 19

Valproic acid, 17
Volume of distribution (V_D), 19.
  See also Distribution of drugs
  definition of, **21**